The Practice of
Primary Nursing
Second Edition

Relationship-Based,
Resource-Driven Care Delivery

Marie Manthey, MNA, FAAN, FRCN

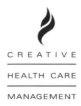

CREATIVE

HEALTH CARE

MANAGEMENT

The Practice of Primary Nursing, Second Edition
Copyright © 2002 by Marie Manthey

ISBN 13: 978-1-886624-17-7

Seventh Printing: April 2008

11 10 09 08   10 9 8 7

For permission and ordering information, write to:

CREATIVE
HEALTH CARE
MANAGEMENT

Creative Health Care Management, Inc.
1701 American Blvd. East, Suite 1
Minneapolis, MN 55425

chcm@chcm.com
or call: 800.728.7766 or 952.854.9015
www.chcm.com

This book is dedicated to Florence Marie Fisher, a nurse who cared for me when I was hospitalized at the age of five with scarlet fever, in St. Joseph's Hospital, Chicago. Although I never saw her again, her personalized and very humane care of me became a model I have followed throughout my life and professional career. This dedication is also made to all those nurses who recognize the profound influence this special kind of nursing practice can have on the lives of their patients and who, by practicing it themselves, perpetuate the proud tradition and invaluable legacy of all of the nurses like Ms. Fisher ultimately the highest tribute of all.

Contents

Foreword

I consider it a pleasure to review Marie Manthey's book, *The Practice of Primary Nursing*, and an honor to be asked to write a foreword.

I first met Marie Manthey when she visited me at Good Samaritan Hospital in Phoenix, Arizona. She was then at the University of Minnesota Health Sciences Center, working on the implementation of Primary Nursing on one of the units. I can remember her enthusiasm and excitement when she described what she was doing. During the intervening years I have had occasion to hear Marie at meetings; and she spent a day at Vanderbilt offering a workshop on Primary Nursing.

I believe Primary Nursing is more important today in the hospital than it was when Marie started it. This book is important because it takes us through the changes in the profession from a historical perspective to why Primary Nursing is essential—not only from the patient's point of view but by putting the accountability for nursing care where it must lie—with the staff nurse. The increasing job satisfaction is essential.

From a nursing service administrator's point of view I have worked with staff through various organizational arrangements of delivering nursing care at the unit level. None were Primary Nursing and none were really successful.

"That's the way nursing should really be" is what I have heard from staff nurses when they discuss Primary Nursing.

As one of many nursing service administrators in the country I believe there are three essentials to consider in managing a nursing department: (1) individualized nursing care for the patient, (2) increasing the awareness amongst staff nurses that they are accountable to the patient for their nursing care, and (3) appropriate utilization of the staff nurse. If the latter is not nursing, she is not being utilized appropriately.

I believe that Marie's book is long overdue and will have a significant impact upon the practice of nursing in the United States. I am delighted to have had the opportunity to review the book and to write this introduction.

Rosamond Gabrielson
Vanderbilt Medical Center
Nashville, Tennessee

Ingeborg G. Mauksch

Foreword

Contemporary nursing literature abounds with thoughtful descriptions and even definitions or problems besetting the profession: its low status, its economic plight, its lack of prestige, its powerlessness, its exclusion from the significant decision-making processes, and its lack of control over its own practice. Marie Manthey's book represents a "first" because it addresses a focal problem of nursing care delivery; it defines it as the delivery of nursing care in a bureaucratic organization and then provides a solution in the form of Primary Nursing. Significantly, this solution also touches on some of the other problems of the profession, thus demonstrating that Primary Nursing is not only a system of nursing care delivery, but also a source of new opportunities to achieve behaviors which are necessary to deal with these other problems.

Primary Nursing as defined and described by Manthey truly represents a system of nursing care delivery. It is a holistic model which consists of policies, procedures, relationships, behaviors, attitudes and competencies. Manthey substantiates this by pointing out that a system of care delivery encompasses a service to people and thus must evidence the characteristics necessary to meet the needs of consumers beyond the customary therapeutic and supportive interventions. In order to achieve this, nurses must be provided with an environment which allows them to attain a sense of egalitarianism *vis a vis* other health care providers, notably physicians. Further, this environment must offer them the opportunity to engage in participatory management in the nursing arena rather than continue to force them to function in the traditional authoritarian structure still mainly prevalent in hospitals, and thus in nursing departments.

Participation in management in turn, Manthey postulates, gives the nurse an opportunity to share in the decisions which she then carries out. This process enables her to develop much needed confidence in her competence, so that she can establish herself as a professional who indeed has the expertise necessary to deliver nursing care of high quality and finally to replace the long pursued submissive woman's role with that of an autonomous person. Once this change in autonomy has been accomplished, we are told, the nurse can move towards the exercise of authority which is necessary to control her professional practice.

The Practice of Primary Nursing will have a major and much needed impact upon the hospital as an institution. Manthey perceptively stresses the need for the hospital and its functionaries to become more humane and more people-oriented. She believes that this system of nursing care delivery can serve as a catalyst to bring about this change, and also to be an instrument in this change process.

For a long time now there has been an ongoing struggle between professional and bureaucratic values in the hospital. Primary nursing confronts this struggle, and suggests a constructive way of accommodating it. If nursing's accommodation is successful, it seems logical to assume that this system of accommodation will also assist other professional practices who experience a similar struggle in the hospital to deal with it. Manthey does not claim to be the originator of all of these ideas, nor does she believe that Primary Nursing will solve the myriad of the hospital's problems. But she quite justifiably maintains that Primary Nursing does exemplify nursing's purpose, and that it does indeed represent a system of delivery which enables nurses to practice professionally in the hospital, and to maximize their contribution to patient care.

As one greatly concerned with the future, I value this book. Primary Nursing constitutes the future of nursing practice, and thus represents a significant resource for today's students whose practice will shape the reality of nursing in the future. This book offers the nursing student an analysis of care delivery in the hospital which should assist her in the formulation of a role consistent with her professionalism and with her newfound egalitarianism in the world of tomorrow's health care. And finally, perhaps most significantly, Primary Nursing provides a system of care to the patient which he has long deserved and badly needed. Professional services are meaningful only if they meet societal needs. Patient care in hospitals has not done this for a long time, if ever. Primary Nursing offers the vehicle to accomplish this service to the society. Let us hope its promise will be realized.

Ingeborg G. Mauksch
Vanderbilt School of Nursing
Nashville, Tennessee

June Werner, RN, MN, MSN, CNAA

Foreword

Primary Nursing at Evanston

In 1971 I became chair of the Evanston (IL) Hospital Department of Nursing. I had set up eleven conditions of employment related to the expectations of the Evanston community and of the finest nurses I knew. The administrative staff accepted my conditions. I was known to the nursing staff since the year before I had developed and taught a course designed for the management of care for nurse managers.

Within two months, the leadership staff had stabilized and committed to our goal. However, we were still using a team nursing model to deliver care. We regularly asked how we could do things better.

About this time, *Nursing Forum* ran an article by Marie Manthey briefly presenting the Primary Nursing model. The goal of Primary Nursing is to empower and support nurses and to provide clinically competent, humane, individualized care to patients and their families.

This idea seemed worth exploring. We sent two of the leadership staff to Minneapolis to observe Marie's model. We also explored two other approaches, but decided that Primary Nursing would best meet the needs of our patients and staff. Our observers shared their findings from Minneapolis with the Nursing Executive Council where the idea was met with skepticism. Responses ranged from "too idealistic," and "the doctors would never stand for it," to "impossible to implement." Although the attractiveness of the model was indisputable Nursing Executive Council members felt they could not support it.

We decided to continue considering Primary Nursing. We asked ourselves, "What would it take to develop a pilot program?" A kind of destiny played into our plan. We learned that the significant other of one of our administrative residents was visiting from Minneapolis. She was not only a nurse, but a Primary Nurse at Miller Hospital, where the model was under way.

We called a special luncheon meeting to meet with this nurse. The result was magical. She explained how the model worked, the role and function of Primary Nurses, the relationships that formed between the Primary Nurse and the patients and families, and the freedom the Primary Nurse had to address the quality of life of the patient and family. Our guest from Minneapolis was so motivated and so enriched by this new way to practice. She won us over.

We started to work diligently to prepare for the pilot project. First, we made certain that the 500-plus physicians were exposed to the expected changes. We had many early morning coffee and donut meetings with various Medical Services. In retrospect, we decided that one large, well-focused cocktail party would have been more efficient.

The Pilot Unit required a competent, experienced head nurse. It had to have at least 50 per cent RN staff and patients in at least three services. We chose a medical unit with oncology, hematology and pulmonary patients. We developed an orientation to Primary Nursing and worked with the staff to prepare them for the changes. On Valentine's Day, 1972 we initiated the pilot program. We decided on reasonable patient and family outcomes with a very attentive support system.

Despite the best-laid plans, we had glitches. The head nurse we selected was "put to bed" with a "tentative pregnancy." This required identifying, orienting and supporting an appropriate alternative leader. Tragedy occurred when a number of staff enroute from a colleague's wedding, had an automobile accident with injuries. This caused a considerable amount of absence during the first ten days. But the unit was undaunted, and continued working through the crisis.

The physicians' reaction to Primary Nursing was mixed. Some had difficulty with primary nurses who knew more about their patients than they did. Others welcomed a high level of clinical competence of their patients' Primary Nurse. One patient who knew she was going to die shared her concerns with her Primary Nurse. She wanted the doctor to tell her husband of her prognosis, but since the physician had never discussed the issue with her, she had difficulty raising the subject. The Primary Nurse spoke with the patient's attending physician, who seemed uncomfortable at the prospect of such a foreboding conversation. The Primary Nurse assured the physician that she would be there with him and raise the subject appropriately. The conversation went as planned. The patient was relieved and the husband was grief stricken but now could be comforted while he himself could comfort and support his wife.

We have many similar examples in which Primary Nurses acted as a bridge between their patients and physicians. These were often specialists who had not seen the patient until the admission.

Toward the end of the pilot project, a highly respected oncologist came to my office with a problem. It had become clear that the growing oncology service needed more private rooms for reverse isolation. Members of that service wanted their patients cared for by Primary Nurses. "Could we please have that model service in the new unit?" queried this gentle concerned physician. I explained that it had taken us two months of concentrated preparation for the pilot unit.

The nursing leadership staff met to consider expediting the training. We bargained for six weeks. In spite of incredible effort, nurses were not yet comfortable with this practice model. The physicians, however, so appreciated this "partnership" with their patients' nurses that this improved communication carried the practice. The head nurse, by now called clinical coordinator, was a paragon of clinical virtue and had been skeptical from the beginning. In the end, it was the medical staff that convinced her that this continuity would be successful in improving care. Greater satisfaction for patients, nurses and physicians would result. In a short time, this clinical coordinator—who herself carried a small case load of primary patients—became one of our most accomplished Primary Nurses.

The Pilot Project was scheduled to come to an end over the summer for evaluation. The staff knew this. These nurses asked to meet with the Nursing leadership staff before the summer vacation. The staff informed us that they did not want to discontinue Primary Nursing. They wanted our approval for a plan that, though imperfect, would maintain the Primary Nursing model. Together, we developed some ground rules: No nurses would work on that unit unless they had experience in our Primary Nursing model. We would keep a journal of the highs and lows of the experience. It was the enthusiasm, commitment and intellectual and emotional energy of these nurses that convinced us.

In mid-spring I had been invited by University of Indiana, Indianapolis School of Nursing to give a presentation on Primary Nursing. Several Primary Nurses, the clinical coordinator, the continuing education staff and I went to discuss the history and development, working with the medical staff, the administration, and other aspects of Primary Nursing.

When the presentation was over, Joyce Clifford, soon to be appointed Nursing Director at Beth Israel Hospitals in Boston, asked if she and some of her staff could come to Evanston to see Primary Nursing in action.

Several week later, Joyce arrived on a Saturday, unannounced and accompanied by colleagues, to see what happens to Primary Nursing on a weekend. She called me quite apologetically on Monday. She admitted that she had been skeptical, but felt that if Primary Nursing worked on weekends, it would be viable any time. Joyce became a great proponent of Primary Nursing. Beth Israel Hospital became first a laboratory and then a showcase for Primary Nursing.

Once we got Primary Nursing established in Evanston, it became well known throughout the hospital and community. The Nursing Leadership asked clinical coordinators to "apply" for support to initiate Primary Nursing on their unit, after meeting several criteria. During this time, while the Chicago area experienced a nursing shortage, we rarely had a vacancy. A national company, conducting a nurse survey was surprised to find our nurse satisfaction among the highest in the country, in spite of our median level salaries.

By the spring of 1975, we had developed a goal that by July patients being admitted should also be informed who his or her Primary Nurse was. While the physician was responsible for their medical needs, each patient would have a designated Primary Nurse responsible for his or her nursing care. Each Primary Nurse carried a defined caseload, developing a one-on-one relationship with their patients and their families. Primary Nursing Associates were designated to care for the patient and relate to the family when the Primary Nurse was off duty. The Evanston community was ready for this.

As we expected, almost always Primary Nurses and patients' Primary Physicians created a viable collaborative relationship. In the late 1980's, the president of the medical staff announced that our litigation rate for physicians was less than one-third of the Illinois average. A round of enthusiastic applause took over the auditorium. As the applause subsided, Dr. Vick admitted that they were clearly a fine group of physicians. However, he added, the lower litigation rate was, in addition, clearly a reflection of the high level of clinical competence of the nursing staff and the fact that Primary Nurses had become a partner in patient care. "Those nurses," he said, "kept the communication open with patients, their families and their physicians." As a result, physicians became nursing's greatest supporters.

The Evanston community became very much aware of the advantages of Primary Nursing. Mothers come to Evanston to have their babies, and often requested the Primary Nurse "we had the last time." Primary Nurses went to their patients' memorial services and supported families in arranging for bereavement counseling. The Continuity of Care Department negotiated discharge planning and when necessary, also made it possible for a patient's Primary Nurse to make a home visit and, if the patient was readmitted, to be assigned the same primary nurse.

I have never experienced a system where nurses were so committed to the quality of life of the patients and their families.

In one memorable incident, my husband and I were driving across town to the memorial service of one of his colleagues who had endured many admissions to Evanston Hospital. My husband was gently chiding me for "working too hard." I agreed to review my work life. The memorial service was inspiring and substantive. Toward the end, the patient's widow introduced family members and then the Primary Nurse. She explained how important the Primary Nurse had been, working on behalf of the patient and his family. It was a fitting, highly public tribute to our Primary Nursing Model and to the Primary Nurse, who was a clinically skilled, responsive advocate for the patient and his family. After the service, my husband said, "I can see that it's worth whatever it takes."

Morale of nurses and nursing units was high. We began to receive community acknowledgment. We became an official Magnet hospital and were cited by JCAHO for nursing excellence. I received the National League of Nursing's Jean McVicar award for Excellence and Creativity in Nursing. I accepted this honor on behalf of the nurses in the Evanston Hospital Corporation who made this happen. This time was, in the words of Emily Hollenberg, our Camelot.

Starting in the late 1980s a tremendous amount of attention was paid to "the bottom line." Some saw Primary Nursing as a "Cadillac" nursing model. These administrators maintained this misconception despite evidence that the Evanston Hospital Corporation's nursing costs were lower than other teaching hospitals. The physicians pleaded with the administration to keep the Primary Nursing model in place. Nevertheless, nursing was to be restructured and become an administrative department rather than a clinical one. Many physicians and hospital leaders felt that nursing had become "too powerful."

In the ensuing struggle, the leadership changed. I resigned. Ninety percent of the clinical coordinators left. The quality of care as perceived by the physicians and the community drastically diminished. The Evanston Hospital Corporation has since experienced critical nursing shortages and a deteriorating reputation in the community.

There is more than one lesson to be learned here. The most important may be that an actualized commitment to safe, effective, humane care of patients and their families, consistently applied by competent professionals and support staff will benefit everyone—including the public image of the institution.

Here is the list of the architects of Primary Nursing in the Evanston Hospital System and those who supported its evolution, the staff who nurtured it to a mature, humane, successful professional model: Rhonda Anderson, Joann Appleyard, Selma Arp, Karen Barnes, Olga Church, Bernadette Dominguez, Sue Driscol, Rita Garber, Sue Gulianelli, Emily Hollenberg, Mark Peletier, Irene Pierce, Ann Porter, Linda Rasmusen, Karen Ringle, Nancy Semerdjian, Jane Stenski, and Norma Tribble.

June Werner, RN, MN, MSN, CNAA

Foreword

Primary Nursing at Beth Israel Hospital

As I write this reminiscence of Primary Nursing, I realize that it is more than thirty years since I was introduced to this nursing model that has become almost synonymous with professional nursing practice. I was teaching nursing administration in the graduate program of Indiana University in Indianapolis, when I was asked to facilitate a presentation featuring Evanston Hospital and June Werner, then chair of nursing of that suburban Chicago hospital. June and her staff were presenting the new nursing care delivery system they had piloted in their quest for improving the way nurses provided care to hospitalized patients. I had just become convinced that service settings needed to implement more of the organizing elements inherent in small work groups. As I listened to June and her staff talk about this model of care—one that promoted the individual nurse rather than the group—I must admit my skepticism abounded. I had been away from practice for about two years and my lack of practical experience with Primary Nursing and inability to find much about it in the literature made be wonder if this could really become a wide-spread and successful system for nursing care delivery. Yet, parts of this model resonated with the work of Lydia Hall, a nurse leader whom I much admired. In the early 1960s, she experimented with changing the way registered nurses were assigned direct services to patients. From my own experience with Lydia Hall's work, I had experimented with reorganizing unit-based nursing services while at the University of Alabama in Birmingham. Using "group practices", we tried to keep nurses with the same groups of patients and physicians. I believed strongly that improved continuity would better achieve the essential communication required for safe care.

But these efforts did not compare with the total re-organization in this model of care demonstrated by the Evanston Hospital nursing staff. I learned that the model was an extension of the work of Marie Manthey and colleagues at the University of Minnesota Hospitals and soon found the scant literature available in 1972. Yet I remained somewhat skeptical about the realities of implementing a system based on Marie's descriptions and trials on one unit at Evanston Hospital.

My attention was quickly turned to the overwhelming needs I found at Beth Israel Hospital in the fall of 1973. Dissatisfaction with nursing care was expressed by all—patients, families, doctors, administrators and particularly nurses. Turnover was high, and morale low. The need for change was immediate. In no way did my thinking begin with Primary Nursing. Indeed, there were so many improvements needed that a model such as Primary Nursing seemed out of reach. Our job was to concentrate on how to improve patient care and nurse job satisfaction.

So began the history of Primary Nursing at the Beth Israel Hospital in Boston. As we examined the opportunities and system barriers for improved care and nursing satisfaction, the elements of Primary Nursing surfaced again and again—continuity, caregiver-to-caregiver communication, decision-making and accountability among them. Excitement abounded about the changing role of the registered nurse responsible for completing the tasks associated with care to that of planning and evaluating the care of the patient. As a recognized member of the team, registered nurses were now positioned to use utilize their knowledge and skills more fully

As patients, families and physicians responded positively to the changes in in-patient nursing, RNs in the operating rooms, emergency service and ambulatory settings in particular began seeking elements of Primary Nursing to incorporated into their own practice. We began to understand that the underlying principles of Primary Nursing were more than the design of a nursing assignment or delivery system. They represented the conceptual framework for professional nursing practice. The Beth Israel was, perhaps, the first to incorporate these elements throughout the hospital, across all practice settings—including home care and community health centers—and to establish them as expectations of a professional practice. The model remained intact until 1996.

The principles of Primary Nursing make me feel encouraged about the ability of nurses to continue the important work Marie and her associates began thirty years ago. Primary Nursing is a value-driven system of care delivery. It focuses on the nurse-patient relationship and the important components of communication and continuity essential for safe practice. It promotes the natural role of nurses as coordinators of care, an increasingly critical role in today's fast paced and complex health system. Primary Nursing encourages care planning with other professionals, which is essential in building team-based care-delivery systems.

Patient safety, a major focus for today's health agencies, was considered to have improved substantially with the continuity of Primary Nursing. And a number of studies suggested that Primary Nursing was no more expensive than other delivery models, and might actually cost less. In sum, this system holds many possibilities for health systems that are interested in better patient outcomes and customer satisfaction, more efficient use of resources and reductions in errors. Primary Nursing is indeed the practice model best suited for the future.

Joyce C. Clifford, RN, PhD, FAAN
Executive Director
Institute for Nursing Health Care Leadership

Nancy Moore, PhD, RN

Foreword

I am convinced that the chaos we are experiencing in health care will settle down when we truly focus on the patient.

Marie Manthey

I first met Marie Manthey during a conference, *A Staffing Crisis: Nurse/Patient Ratios*, during the summer of 2000. As I listened to her talk, I heard words that resonated with my soul and, I believe, the soul of nursing. She spoke of relationship-centered and resource-based care. She reminded us that we must look at resources in the context of patient needs, that the prioritization and delivery of care is part of the contract that nurses have with patients. The public expects nurses to make decisions about care. That is what nurses are licensed to do.

Too often, prioritization is viewed as an ordering of tasks by importance from the nurses' point of view. Little wonder that nurses go home shift after shift and day after day frustrated and angry that they could not meet all of their patients' needs. As I listened I understood that the key to true prioritization—drawing a line separating what will and will not be done—needs to exist in the relationship with the patient. A truly therapeutic relationship exists when the nurse establishes a connection with the patient by asking what needs he or she would like the nurse to address for the day and for the hospital stay. To attempt to prioritize resources without a relationship and knowledge of the patient's needs from the patient's perspective is foolish and perhaps dangerous. Nurses need to refocus on the relationship with the patient.

A plethora of research shows the value of open communication and relationships in health care. Perhaps more important, patients have been telling us for years, "I want a relationship with my nurse, my care provider; and I want a voice in my care. I want one person who knows me and my needs and uses this information for a plan of care that everyone respects and follows."

Although relationships are requisite to effective care and healing, aside from Primary Nursing, formal acknowledgment of their importance in the design of our care models is scant. Similarly, there is also little focus on efforts to help students and practitioners learn to develop effective relationships in the practical realities of health care.

In January, 1992, the Pew Health Professions Commission and the Fetzer Institute began examining ways to promote an integrated approach to health care that affirms the interaction of biomedical and psycho-social factors in health. Targeting health professionals' curricula, the task force conclusion focused on one issue of critical importance: how to enhance and enrich the relationships that are relevant to health care through both education and practice. Relationships are the medium for the exchange of information, feelings and concerns. Relationships are the foundation for the plan of care, an essential ingredient in the satisfaction of patient and practitioner as well as positive health outcomes.

Furthermore, traditional hospitals and financial institutions are validating this growing awareness. The Health Forum of the American Hospital Association, The Healthcare Forum Foundation, Arthur Andersen, and DYG conducted the nationwide study, *Leadership for a Healthy 21st Century* (1999). They concluded that the "age of relationships" best captures the scope of change made possible and inevitable in the modern economy. It is a combination of relationships and the intangible value they generate, combined with traditional assets, that create the foundation for health care and the solution to its challenges.

At Cascade Health Services we are guided by the Healing Health Care Philosophy ethic of healing ourselves, our relationships, our communities. Our intention is to create an environment that supports healing: healing for our patients, their families and caregivers. We understand that a truly healing environment will exist only to the extent that the caregivers themselves have found healing. Healing for each of us is enhanced when we care for ourselves and our team members as well as the people we serve. We are a human service. Who we are and how we work together are what our patients and their families receive. We recognize that healing is enhanced in caring relationships.

This philosophy is congruent with nursing theorist Jean Watson's transpersonal caring nursing science. Watson views nursing as consisting of transpersonal caring actions to protect, enhance and preserve humanity by helping a person find meaning in illness, suffering, pain and experience. Nursing's role is to help the person gain self-knowledge, control and self-healing wherein a sense of inner harmony is restored.

We view Primary Nursing as the prototype for a care delivery system that addresses the importance of relationships in health care. Primary Nursing has endured for decades for good reasons. Primary nursing provides a system for building-in the nurse-patient relationship. This relationship is the vehicle for transpersonal caring, as well as professional judgment. It is this relationship that allows nurses to appropriately allocate their energy resource in the patient's best interest. Also, we are convinced that the therapeutic relationship is the key to nurses finding meaning in their work, thus revitalizing nursing. It is through the individual responsibility-relationship of the nurse with the patient that the values of caring and healing that we treasure will be realized for the patient and the nurse.

Yes, Marie Manthey: I, too, am convinced that the chaos we are experiencing in health care will settle down when we truly focus on the patient.

Nancy Moore, PhD, RN
Healing Health Services Vice President
Cascade Health Services
Bend, Oregon

Preface

This book is written for anyone who wants to know about Primary Nursing. It is not meant to be the last word on the subject, nor is it the first. I have tried to be clear in writing about this system, because the system itself is very simple. However, because it is not also easy, there is a tendency to make it seem more complex than it is. In my efforts to honor the beauty of its simplicity, some may feel I have ignored or slighted important complex related issues. I prefer to err in favor of simplicity, but have tried to deal thoroughly with every issue of *immediate importance to the system*. If there are complex issues I have not dealt with adequately in this book it is because I do not feel they are central to Primary Nursing. Everything is related to everything else in this world, so many lines have to be drawn and mine have been drawn rather tightly around the system of Primary Nursing.

Primary Nursing is a delivery system designed: 1) to allocate twenty-four-hour responsibility for each patient's care to one individual nurse, and 2) to assign this nurse the actual provision of her patient's physical care whenever possible. The Primary Nurse leaves information and instructions for her patient's care when she is off duty, so the nurse who relieves her knows about the patient as a person and exactly how care should be administrated in this particular case. The Primary Nurse also has major responsibility for preparing the patient and/or his family for discharge.

Primary Nursing is a system for delivering nursing care in an inpatient facility; that is *all* it is. It is not a solution to the problem of the difference between "professional" and "technical" levels of practice and preparation; it is not a solution to the issue created by the use of LPNs in acute care settings. It will not solve staffing problems caused by an inadequate budget, nor will it increase the workload. (So budgets should not be expanded in the name of Primary Nursing!) It will solve neither personnel management nor inter-personal relationship problems. It is a system originally designed for delivering nursing care to sick people who are hospitalized. It was developed on a real station in a real hospital during a period of serious nurse-power shortage. The staff was not hand-picked, nor was it considered unusually qualified. Thus, the system is designed for maximum use of *available* resources. No additional money was allocated from any source during the development phase. It is an innovation that works in the real world because that is the crucible in which it was originally developed and tested.

High quality nursing care should be the goal of every nurse, educator and manager. High quality nursing to me means care that is individualized to a particular patient, administered humanely and competently, comprehensively and with continuity. Primary Nursing is one means of accomplishing that quality of care. It may not be the only way to do so; it is the proven way with which this book concerns itself.

The first part of the book (Chapters One and Two) explains the recent history of nursing as I understand it to have impacted on the present. I have started with a historical analysis because during ten years of teaching nurses about this system the historical approach has proved to be the most effective way to prepare them to receive the new information with minimum rejection. An understanding of how we got where we are helps people avoid becoming defensive about their current situations and opens them to forward motion or a growth experience. To understand why Primary Nursing was developed in the first place, it has been helpful to describe, graphically at times, the problems staff nurses, patients and others experience in using other delivery systems, notably "team nursing." Since many people are still struggling mightily to make team nursing work, an understanding of its development from an historical perspective reduces the emotional negativism such a critique can cause.

Primary Nursing evolved from an effort to improve on the implementation of team nursing so that high quality nursing could be effectively achieved. The problems with team nursing as they were experienced in that setting were identified and attempts were made to correct those problems without changing the system. Those efforts failed, so an alternative delivery system was designed. That system was called Primary Nursing. The three problems identified with team nursing were: 1) fragmentation of care; 2) complex channels of communication; and 3) shared responsibility. Recognition of these in turn provided the bases of Primary Nursing. Thus the basic elements, the strengths of Primary Nursing, as described in Chapter Three, are the result of growth and learning from team nursing.

Chapter Four, The Implementation of Primary Nursing, is the backbone of this book. In this chapter I have tried to explain how to implement this system successfully based on all the experience I have had doing so in the past ten years. The recommendations for implementation which I make are a result of what I learned as I implemented the concept and what I learned from the efforts of others using different approaches.

My observations and conclusions are a product of my values and beliefs about mankind. I am an equalitarian with strong anti-elitist prejudices. I believe that mankind and womankind are good and that people want to do the right thing; thus, I have a great deal of confidence in the integrity of a system designed by the staff members who will use it. I truly believe that a system so implemented will provide an effective way to deliver high quality care. Thus, my recommendations about implementation focus intensely on staff member involvement in the implementation process.

Re-humanization of hospital care is the goal that has been my strongest motivation. Decentralized decision making seems to me to be the organizational framework within which humane treatment of the sick can most effectively be provided and maintained. In order for the patient to be treated humanely, the staff who deliver the care must be treated humanely by the management of the institution. Decentralized decision-making is an organizational framework wherein authority for decision making is delegated downward in the institution to the level of action to which, in nursing, is the bedside. By authorizing the staff, who deliver care, to decide how that care will be delivered, the institution recognizes that the staff are intelligent and educated human beings whose intellects can be used in deciding how to provide sensitive and sensible individualized care. Decentralized decision making recognizes the inherent worth of the intelligence each employee can bring to care of the patients. Patients cannot receive humane and thoughtful care from staff members who have been treated in a dehumanized fashion by their managers.

Management responsibilities in a decentralized decision making structure are clearly different from those in a centralized, authoritarian structure. One of the most obvious differences is that the thrust of management in a decentralized setting is facilitative rather than directive. In Primary Nursing implementation, the change process should be dominated by the staff nurses. The decision to put the Primary Nursing system into effect must be made at the staff nurse level. Otherwise, decentralized decision making has not been experienced by the staff nurses and cannot be successfully used in the clinical decision making required by the system.

Occasionally, staff nurses resent this implementation style. As a director of nursing I have had staff nurses beg me to tell them what to do, but these are a very small minority of very immature people (of all ages). Most staff nurses eagerly accept the challenge of self-determination and the resulting growth experiences are thrilling to see and profound to feel.

This approach to implementation reflects my deep belief that it is time for nursing to grow up and for staff nurses to stop acting like and being treated like little children. Most staff nurses I have met are mature people. Many have dealt with significant life events and accept heavy life responsibilities. Yet, at work, they are called "girls," treated like children and made to feel like "just a staff nurse" (a phrase that is sickeningly similar to "just a housewife"). The implementation process I recommend gives all staff members an opportunity to use legitimately rights they have always possessed but seldom felt free to use openly.

Nurses need to develop an appreciation for the reality of legitimate authority. Many nurses have been made to feel that because the physician controls medical treatment and the hospital administrator defines the mission and policies of the hospital that these two traditionally male dominated functions also have authority and control over all aspects of nursing practice. If a director of nursing is to be held liable for the quality of care that is administered by the nursing staff, she must have authority to set the standards of care and introduce appropriate delivery systems. This *authority* is legitimately hers by virtue of the *responsibility* she has accepted.

Many directors have asked me how I got the physicians or the hospital administrator to let me do Primary Nursing. The simplest and most honest answer is "I didn't ask them; I told them." Since Primary Nursing usually does not cost any more money in salary dollars, permission, so to speak, from the hospital administrator is not necessary. However, in introducing the concept it is extremely important that all key members of the institution understand the changes being made. In so informing them, however, the director of nursing needs to be aware of the fact that neither the physicians nor the administrator have legitimate authority to tell her what nursing system is appropriate for the nursing staff to use. If that were their job, they could save the cost of the director's salary.

This book is about Primary Nursing: how it developed, what it is and how to implement it. It is also a book about power, self-determination and the humanization of hospital care. Primary Nursing is not really a new idea. It is a logical approach to caring for sick people the way *we* would like to be cared for if *we* were sick. However, the process of returning to these simple values is revolutionary in that it represents a reallocation of power…from a faceless, anonymous, hierarchical, authoritarian bureaucracy to the staff nurse who is responsible for the care of a sick person.

It should be noted that staff nurses have been referred to throughout the text as "she" and sick persons as "he." The use of the feminine pronoun for nurses comes easily and naturally, but even though I am proud that nursing has historically been a woman's profession I have not intentionally discriminated against male colleagues. The she/he, nurse/patient pairing is simply a matter of convenience adopted purely for the sake of the reader.

Primary Nursing Revisited

This second edition of *The Practice of Primary Nursing* preserves the integrity of the story told in the first edition. The story of the first ten years of Primary Nursing's development is as true now as it was then. This new edition contains an addendum to each chapter reflecting my thoughts and experiences today. In other words, a continuation of the story told in the first edition.

Twenty years have passed since *The Practice of Primary Nursing* was originally published. Primary Nursing revolutionized our thinking about hospital nursing practice in the United States and around the world. *The Practice of Primary Nursing* was written long after the original implementation, and only after I had figured out to my own satisfaction the organizational implications of the concept and developed a successful implementation method. After carefully reviewing the first edition, I concluded that, in the main, after more than twenty years of experience, the original text still reflects the principles and processes involved in implementing Primary Nursing, a professional practice care delivery system. I believe it stands as the "classic" description.

However, because of changes in health care and the things I've learned along the way, I want to change or emphasize certain points that have evolved since the book's original publication. The second edition is based on real-world experiences implementing care delivery systems throughout the United States, as well as in other countries. In this way, readers will not only have access to the "classic," but also to how changes in health care and my own learning and growth have influenced my thinking about the delivery of professional nursing care, particularly within the acute care arena.

Acknowledgments

The number of people whose help in preparing this book should really be acknowledged is boundless. Ever since Primary Nursing was first implemented I have had innumerable opportunities to meet and talk with nurses all over the country and from each I have learned and grown.

A special expression of gratitude to those members of the administration of the University of Minnesota Hospitals who, not without taking considerable risks, provided the fertile environment in which Primary Nursing was first developed. John Westerman, Hospital Administrator, and Florence Julian, Director of Nursing, were especially supportive, as was my partner in heading the pilot project, David Preston, and the first head nurse, Diane Bartels. Needless to say, the encouragement and support of the entire nursing staff was both invaluable and appreciated beyond measure.

I would like to thank my typist, Pat Moore, for help of a more concrete nature, and my children Claire and Mark, for help of a more subtle nature. They have helped and supported me at crucial points in my development and I can only hope that I have similarly helped them.

The Practice of
Primary Nursing

Relationship-Based,
Resource-Driven Care Delivery

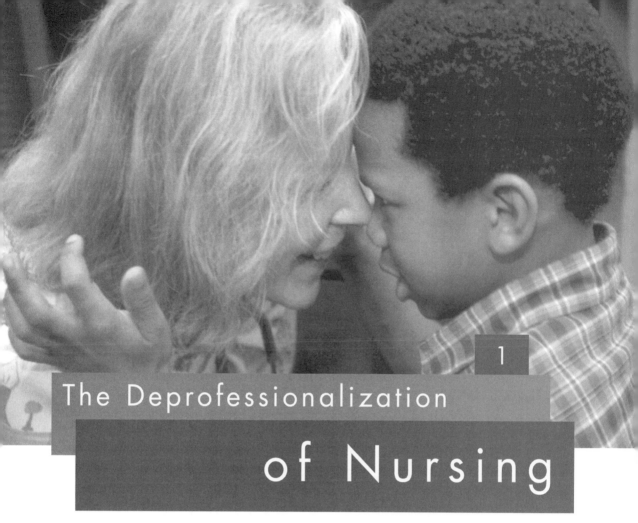

The Deprofessionalization
of Nursing

Primary Nursing is a delivery system for nursing at the station level that facilitates professional nursing practice despite the bureaucratic nature of hospitals. The practice of any profession is based on an independent assessment of a client's needs which determines the kind and amount of service to be rendered: services in bureaucracies are usually delivered according to routine pre-established procedures without sensitivity to variations in needs. In bureaucracies, functions are grouped into bureaus or departments, headed by chiefs who usually retain decision-making authority. Thus, for professionals to exist in a bureaucracy, the system used to deliver the services must be designed to minimize the bureaucratic impact and maximize the value of their individualized services.

Within a bureaucracy, many different delivery systems may coexist to accomplish the many different functions of the various departments. These systems can enhance and facilitate either bureaucratic or professional values depending on the nature of the services rendered and the design of the system. Before Primary Nursing was established at the University of Minnesota in 1969, the delivery system used for hospital nursing reflected bureaucratic rather than professional values. Both functional nursing (in which one nurse passes all medications, another does all treatments and several people give all baths) and the team nursing systems are designed according to a mass production model of service delivery; the least complex tasks are assigned to the least trained workers, the more complex to more skilled workers and so on up a hierarchy of task complexity. In those systems, registered nurses are assigned two functions: 1) to administer the most complex tasks and 2) to coordinate and supervise the tasks done by the lesser prepared workers. Registered nurses in this system are not professional care givers; rather they are checker-uppers of cheaper-doers. Primary Nursing is a delivery system that creates the opportunity for nurses to develop a truly professional role in hospital nursing today.

Fifty years ago, when graduate nurses worked in their patients' own homes, there was no need to be concerned about a delivery system for individualized patient care. The nurse took care of the sick person from the time the need for care was identified until it no longer existed; care was personally administered by the nurse according to the assessment she made of the individual needs of the patient. There were no rules or regulations, no routine procedures, no hospital policies, time schedules, or supervisors. She practiced nursing with a degree of independence unheard of in modern hospital nursing.

This type of practice had more of the characteristics sociologists use in describing a profession than does the practice of the modern nurse. It is my contention that despite all the lip service that has been paid to the process of professionalization, nursing has in fact undergone a serious process of *de*professionalization. The change in setting from home to hospital and to the delivery systems subsequently designed for the hospital setting have significantly decreased the professionalism of nursing practice.

During those same fifty years, nurse leaders have labored heroically to upgrade nursing education in the firm belief that higher educational standards elevate professional stature. They changed the setting of education from the hospital, with its apprenticeship training programs, to the college and its classroom programs. Their efforts were successful. The majority of nurse preparation now takes place in educational rather than service settings. It is unfortunate however that the effect of that success on nursing's professional stature has been diminished by the simultaneous deprofessionalization of nursing practice. Primary Nursing is a delivery system that promises to maximize the professional values acquired in these educational programs by facilitating professional role development.

There are four characteristics generally agreed to be sociologists as descriptive of the ways a profession can be differentiated from another endeavor or occupation. These are: 1) an identifiable body of knowledge that can best be transmitted in a formal educational program; 2) autonomy of decision-making; 3) peer review of practice; and 4) identification with a professional organization as the standard setter and arbiter of practice. I believe that the practice of nurses in the twenties contained more of all of these characteristics than did the practice of nurses in the seventies, and that this change in the degree of professionalism is directly attributable to the change in the setting of practice that has occurred over the last fifty years.

A comparison of nursing in the twenties and in the seventies in terms of the four characteristics of a profession illustrates this point.

The *identifiable body of knowledge* that could best be communicated in a formal educational setting was more identifiable in the twenties when Nightingale's *Notes on Nursing* was the basic textbook. Today's variety of generic curriculum theories boggles the mind. Different schools teach nursing using different theoretical frameworks and different skill levels, resulting in confusion and ambiguity about what can be expected of graduate nurses. In the twenties, it was simple; all graduates could fill all nursing needs for all patients! Today, two-year, three-year, and four-year programs prepare nurses to perform different functions with varying levels of competence in ability to make clinical judgments. While the quality of education is undoubtedly superior now, the confusion and ambiguity over the content has so seriously blurred the boundaries of the body of knowledge that it is no longer clearly identifiable.

Autonomy of decision-making is a natural result of acquiring an identifiable body of knowledge, since it follows logically that only those who have acquired this knowledge are qualified to make decisions in that particular field of endeavor. The privilege of decision-making autonomy is based on a clear demarcation of the boundaries of knowledge. Currently, there is much confusion over what nurses know and can do independently. Neither nurses, their patients, nor their colleagues agree about which decisions are appropriately made by a nurse and only a nurse.

In the twenties, the nurse was concerned with the comfort and treatment of the patient and with maintaining the health of the family. The private duty nurse entered the patient's home and took charge of the patient's total care. There was no head nurse to supervise her and no clinical instructor to orient her. She had the authority to decide when and how the physician's treatment orders were carried out. In addition, she educated her patient and the family about measures they could employ to maintain their own health. It was well understood that during a nurse's stay with a family, she would teach members of the household housekeeping methods, germ theory, comprehensive sanitation techniques, and principles of good nutrition and basic health maintenance. These were part of the nurse's defined body of knowledge. She did not expect, nor was she expected, to consult with the physician or anyone else about routine comfort, sanitation, or nutrition.

In addition, the nurse was the community health educator, in competition with no one else for that role. Nurses, especially public health nurses, were often asked to deliver speeches to community civic groups on topics related to care of the sick and maintenance of health. Graduate nurses were taught how to organize material for a speech and how to deliver a public address, both to a live audience as well as over the radio.

This lack of a clearly defined knowledge base is reflected in the current lack of consensus regarding autonomy of decision-making. A staff nurse will often be unable to identify a single decision that is hers and hers alone to make; and if she does, her colleague working by her side cannot be expected to agree. In fact, the only area of agreement regarding nursing's autonomy that this author has consistently found in talking with other nurses is that there is no such thing.

It is no wonder then that the other health professionals involved in the care of the patient are also unable to articulate a single area of decision-making that belongs to nurses. Thus, many physicians feel it is their right and duty to write orders governing all aspects of a patient's care, including routine comfort measures, such as "turn patient every two hours," "back rub at H.S." and "routine oral hygiene in A.M. and at H.S."

Peer review of practice and *identification with a professional organization* were effectively in place in the twenties through the Boards of Registry and Alumnae Associations. Most cities and towns had a Board of Registry comprised of registered nurses. One of the main functions of the Board was the assignment of cases to nurses.

Physicians or patients needing a private duty nurse called the Board, which acted as a clearinghouse for matching up cases with nurses. To be registered with the Board for private duty, a nurse had to be a member in good standing of her school's Alumnae Association. This was not always easy to maintain since involvement in almost any kind of scandal (especially if a newspaper mentioned the nurse's name) would often result in the nurse's name being "stricken from the roles of the graduates." An example, taken from the actual student records of the Connecticut Training School from the end of the last century, tells of a Miss Happy Jane Daniels, who entered the school in 1884 and was graduated in 1886. The footnote on her student record page read as follows:

> In the autumn of 1888 her name was mentioned in the newspaper in the connection of a divorce of Dr. A_____ from his wife. Her name is no longer on our list of graduates. She is married to Dr. A_____ and lives in New Haven.

Another function of the Board was to receive complaints about a nurse's performance for investigation and action, if any was warranted. Since supervision of a nurse's work after graduation was almost nonexistent, the Board functioned similarly to the way local medical societies do today in the performance of "peer review" of practice.

Finally, the Board acted as a standard setter whenever situations occurred for which no precedent had ever been set. Since home care was individualized and unpredictable, it was not uncommon for the Board to act as arbiter in cases where a dispute about the efficacy of a nurse's action existed.

Peer review of practice in the seventies is foreign concept to most nurses. Because of the hierarchical and authoritarian nature of the bureaucracy, evaluation of performance usually flows from superior to inferior rather than from peer to peer. Staff nurses look to their head nurse to tell them how well or how poorly they are doing. Head nurses look to their supervisors and supervisors to their director of nurses. This author clearly remembers, however, that as a staff nurse, I had a very clear idea of which of my colleagues were good nurses and which ones were not. I was better able to evaluate staff nurses when I was one than later when I was head nurse. The evaluation mechanism in place now, however, assumes that people in superior positions have superior knowledge.

Performance evaluations are supposed to reward excellence and maintain a competent staff by weeding out unsafe and incompetent practitioners. Perhaps if the system functioned more effectively, society would not be clamoring so loudly for better accountability mechanisms. However, in response to society's demands for better accountability, quality assurance programs are now being designed which use staff nurses for both setting standards and for evaluating staff nurse performance. Establishment of peer review of practice through staff nurse dominated quality assurance programs will effectively increase the professionalism of nursing practice.

Nursing today suffers from the absence of a single unifying force that has the power to influence significantly the direction in which the health care delivery system moves. Although the American Nurses Association has an ever-increasing impact on legislation, it often lacks support from nurses (both in terms of individual membership, and their active personal support) for the positions it takes on various issues. For a multitude of reasons, nurses today often look to their employing institutions or individuals for leadership on issues affecting role development, health care delivery, standards of nursing practice, and even guidance on moral and ethical issues in which they are involved daily. When nurses were in private duty, the Board of Registry and the Alumnae Association were professional organizations of great significance and power in the life of a nurse. Since nurses become employees of major institutions, no professional organization has had much impact on the life of the individual nurse.

A comparison of the transition from student to graduate in the twenties and the same process as we enter the eighties clearly depicts the effect of both the shifts in setting of education and practice.

Students in the twenties experienced a training program similar to the one developed fifty years earlier by Florence Nightingale. The Nightingale school emphasized a two-pronged approach to nursing education: 1) The development of exemplary technical skills in treatment measures and facilitating physical comfort and, 2) the development of personal character of impeccable moral purity. Nightingale believed in strict adherence to the rules and regulations promulgated by school authorities to achieve the desired ends. "Deviant " behavior was punished. The emphasis on the development of a "pure" moral character and the use of step-by-step procedures to teach technical skills may have been appropriate to prepare the original nurse pioneers in the 1860's but it did little to prepare the modern woman of the twenties for the variety of situations she faced as an employed private duty nurse.

All aspects of a student's nurse's life were subject to scrutiny and control. On duty, she was expected to carry out all orders from her superiors (both nurse and physicians) with absolute accuracy, military precision, and unquestioning obedience. Off duty, she was expected to lead a life of moral purity; no breath of scandal was permitted to mar the unimpeachable character of a nurse. The superintendent of nurses was concerned with how a student nurse looked, who she spoke to, what she said, how she said it, what she read, what she didn't read, what form of recreation she enjoyed (and with whom), what she ate, and how well she slept. Behavior, which did not measure up to the standard, was met with swift punishment in the form of either a reprimand or dismissal.

The following comments are excerpted from actual student records and reflect typical responses to student performance that deviated from the established procedures. The importance of an attitude of obedience is obvious.

While assisting the night nurse in 2 east showed a disposition to do as she thought best not as she was taught…tested temperature of enemata with her hand…poured solution by sight, not by measure and in other ways was untrustworthy. Reproved but continued as above, dismissed in consequence.

…was severely reprimanded for impertinence to her head nurse…and for insubordination when told if she does any more careless work or is impertinent to anyone or argues with patients or criticizes those in authority she will be dismissed. Left.

…seems in a dream and mind far away…has again been reported as very careless in pouring medicines.

…recorded medicines and treatments before they had been given, including treatment for a patient out on pass. When corrected seems to think that "everyone makes mistakes" …careless, heedless methods. Dismissed.

…was severely reprimanded…she failed to compare a patient's clothing with the list and consequently sent another patient's clothes in the place of the right ones…left the treatment room in an unsatisfactory condition and the package of clothing was pinned together instead of tied. These careless methods if repeated would call for even more severe reprimand.

…left the medicine cabinet standing open, breaking an important rule. Her excuse that she thought another nurse was going to give medicines was not considered sufficient as serious consequences might have followed. She was called to the office and severely reprimanded.

…she is inclined to do things her own way instead of the way she was taught…talks a good deal while about her work…asks questions at inconvenient times…is fond of doing things her own way, but has improved in her manner of taking reproach…failed to carry out orders…was severely reproved and told that the offense would be entered in the records against her…has not improved but rather gone backward…the head nurse dares not leave her in the ward without supervision…she was found very unsatisfactory and dropped [1].

While failing to conform to established procedures was considered a grievous offense, nothing was more serious than conduct viewed as unbecoming a professional nurse. Consider the following examples:

The past three months has not done well…she had been noisy, boisterous, talking in a loud tone of voice. She was reproved for this but in a few weeks other reports were brought to me. She made trouble among the nurses by telling stories and gossiping about them…her conduct on the street and in the Hospital was unprofessional…she went to one of the restaurants with a medical student where liquor was sold but claimed she did not drink any. Dismissed—

…was reprimanded for lingering in the corridor when off duty in the evening. She acknowledged that she was talking with one of the house doctors. Though warned of the consequences, went out one evening with a house doctor, till 1:30 a.m., tried to enter the dormitory through a window. She was called before a special committee and as there could be no extenuation of her conduct, she was expelled from the school.

Dismissed, not up to our standard…would call out of her window to passersby…very familiar with young men about the hospital…undesirable in every way.

Was seen sitting on the floor by the surgical carriage laughing and talking with a patient and another nurse. She was reprimanded for such frivolity and taken from the ward. She violated the most ordinary sense of propriety.

This education did little to prepare a young woman for the challenges and uncertainties she faced as a graduate nurse in private practice. First, there was the uncertainty of the future. If she was on a case, it might last for one day, one week, one month, one year, or longer. However long the duration, the nurse was expected to be on duty all day, every day. A day off could be enjoyed only after a suitable replacement had been located and permission of both the patient and the physician had been secured. When not on a case, the nurse had no assurance whatsoever of whether the next call would come in one day, one week, one month, or never. Thus, from a student life of virtually complete minute-by-minute regulation, the graduate went to a life which alternated between total unpredictability and unremitting constancy. The financial insecurity of this employment situation is obvious.

Another area of uncertainty was the type of equipment and supplies available in the home for use in the care of the patient. The rigid adherence to regulations in the performance of procedures as a student did little to prepare the graduate nurse for the level of innovativeness and adaptability demanded of her in private practice. Some nurses owned a few of the more basic pieces of equipment, but in general the application of comfort measures and treatment procedures required the ability to use everyday household items as sickroom equipment.

The presence or absence of electricity, running water, toilets, bathing facilities, cooking ranges, ice boxes, etc., were factors that significantly affected her practice. The establishment of routine procedures carried over from one household to another was virtually impossible, since, for one thing, electricity and plumbing were just becoming standard household features. Although nothing in her training prepared the nurse to be either flexible or adaptable, the circumstances of care were so variable that case-to-case similarities could not be much relied on.

Finally, the nurse faced untold uncertainties surrounding her ability to establish therapeutic relationships. Nothing in her education prepared her to understand the wide range of behaviors that exist in the real world. The narrowness of her education, particularly the Victorian interpretation of morality, scarcely provided her with a context for understanding human nature. Thus, the ultimate uncertainty she faced was whether or not she would be able to establish and maintain a relationship with the patient and family that would enable her to affect the outcomes of the illness successfully.

Thus, the transition from student nurse to graduate nurse in the twenties was necessarily one of role expansion. Nursing was learned in a setting that was rigid, militaristic, and religiously oriented in an institution governed by rules and regulations dictating all facets of one's work and one's personal life. Nursing was practiced in a setting where differences, variations, unpredictability and uncertainty were the norm and where creativity, adaptability, flexibility and ingenuity were absolute requirements for a successful practice. The system certainly did not guarantee the education of good nurses but, by its very weaknesses, it ensured the "survival of the fittest."

The transition from student nurse to graduate nurse in the seventies was one of role deprivation. Consider the contrast. Education now takes place in institutions of higher education where academic freedom instead of the authority of the superintendent governs curriculum content. Well-prepared faculty design courses to meet objectives which are consistent with the philosophy and theoretical framework of the school. The faculty have a great deal of freedom to choose the appropriate techniques to achieve the educational goals. Students quickly become aware of the level of professional development the faculty has achieved. This awareness initiates the socialization process of the student as a professional using the faculty as role model. Unfortunately, the role modeled is one of professional educator rather than professional nurse, but neither students nor faculty are aware of the importance of the difference. It is one thing to be a successful professional educator in an institution of higher education; it is quite something else to be a successful professional nurse, as a staff nurse in an acute care hospital.

Nursing is no longer taught using a step-by-step procedure approach; as a matter of fact, many schools teach virtually no procedures as such, but rather a process of nursing. Upon graduation, the student enters the health system as staff nurse in an institution that is rule and regulation dominated, where deviations from policy are punishable offenses, and where the word "nursing process" is met by an icy stare. Task accomplishment has high priority in hospital nursing.

Since nursing is now taught in institutions whose primary purpose is teaching "why" rather than "how," the scope of learning is much broader. Liberal arts courses comprise a major component of every generic baccalaureate program; hospital schools and associate degree programs have similarly broadened their scope. Today's students spend short periods of time on the floors, but are exposed to a wide variety of experiences and learning opportunities. They are exposed to a breadth of knowledge unheard of fifty years ago, but to relatively few of the technical skills considered essential in the twenties. In fact, clinical judgment skills, complex techniques, and in some cases, routine comfort measures are considered appropriate "first job" learning experiences. The art and skill of hands-on nursing has thus become an on-the-job learning experience, with economic and sociological ramifications for the profession which have weakened, rather than broadened, it.

Students are taught to provide comprehensive patient care based on a process of nursing using problem-solving skills to develop an individualized plan of care. The case method of patient assignment is used and a student typically cares for one or two patients on any given day. Patients are selected on the basis of a student's learning needs, as perceived by the clinical instructor.

Throughout the education program, freedom of thought and intellectual curiosity are encouraged; kudos are given to students who challenge policies that restrict individualization of care. The bright, inquisitive, aggressive student who challenges established procedures with the innocence of ignorance is cherished by her teachers and rewarded for being courageous and willing to question the establishment. Some see these seekers of truth as the vanguard of a revolutionary force for change that will march forward on graduation days for years to come, prepared to modify the health care delivery system for the good of nursing, and, thus, ultimately for the good of patient care. (If nurses are happy, patient care is bound to be better!)

With the unbounded altruism that typically leads a person into nursing in the first place thus enflamed by the fires of idealism, the new graduate applies for her first staff nurse job in an acute care hospital. As a staff nurse, she finds herself in a position of powerlessness. The job description for her position describes little of what she really does; she may find, however, it can be used to add tasks indiscriminately to her workload. The position of staff nurse is viewed by other professionals in the hospital as the lowest in the pecking order of power. Unfortunately, this attitude is also prevalent in the hierarchy of the many nursing departments where, despite all protestation to the contrary, the attitude of "she's just a staff nurse" is still all too common. Our would-be revolutionary, so recently armed with the weapons of change, finds herself in one of the most powerless positions in the hospital. Her superiors do not expect her to be a change agent; perish the thought. If she can learn what she has to know to do the job, especially how to not "rock the boat," her chances of success and promotion are secure. The speed with which she learns her place will affect how soon she will be rewarded for being a "good nurse."

The modern hospital can still be described in the same language used to describe hospitals in the twenties: militaristic, authoritarian, bureaucratic institutions governed by rules and regulations, called policies and procedures, administered in a structure of authoritarianism that borders on the absolute. The aspiring professional nurse finds herself powerless in a power-dominated system where power rests in the highest positions and only those closest to the seats of power are highly valued. Unfortunately, nothing in her education, including the faculty's professional role modeling, prepared the new nurse to cope successfully with the reality of this powerlessness, let alone to effect change in the face of it.

The problem of role deprivation so aptly described by Marlene Kramer [2] is one of the most devastating problems nursing faces as it comes into the eighties. Thirty percent of the best educated practitioners in nursing change careers within two years of graduation. Our profession is in serious trouble.

The transition from student to graduate in the twenties and in the seventies accurately reflects how the change of practice setting led to the deprofessionalization of nursing. In the twenties, the transition was out of necessity an expansion from a skill-based, narrow education to an independent practice containing many of the characteristics of a profession. By the seventies we find the situation reversed. Broad based, professionally oriented educational programs produce nurses who then go on to fill impotent roles, constricted within rigid sets of rules and regulations. This can be attributed primarily to the change in the setting of practice to the hospital, with its predictably bureaucratic power structure. To regain the element of professionalism nursing once had it is necessary to create a *delivery* system that lives up to the expectations created by contemporary education and facilitates professional practice. That system is Primary Nursing.

Addendum to Chapter One

Deprofessionalization continues to be a major problem, now not only in nursing but within other professions as well. In the last two decades of the 20th century, macro political and economic changes profoundly influenced society, health care and nursing. The two most prominent drivers of change were financial and technological. As capitalism won the "economic war" worldwide, health care in the United States became a business, rather than a social program. For-profit and large HMO-run hospitals, salaried physicians, and elaborate marketing campaigns became the visible signs of system changes in the 1980s and '90s. Competition among hospitals and health care systems drove revenues down, while health care costs overall continued to rise faster than the GNP. Financiers of health care became more and more involved in care decisions, which ultimately reduced the autonomy of physicians and other health professionals. Reimbursement regulations drive clinical decisions, much to the chagrin of physicians and patients. Standardized care protocols and financial/government regulations erode professional autonomy in every allied health discipline. Thus, the deprofessionalization nurses first experienced when their practice moved into hospitals is now being experienced by many professions within and outside the health care system.

Partnering with Patients

Throughout the history of nursing the nurse-patient relationship has been the essence of practice. Primary Nursing resurrected the integrity of that essential partnership in the 1970s, after it had been submerged in bureaucratic controls throughout the post-war period. Although Primary Nursing has been cycling through most nursing departments for nearly thirty years, its very existence—and its practicality—continues to reignite the value of relationship-based practice. This occurs despite the system changes that continuously threaten relationship-based practice within all health professions.

Lack of continuity threatens relationship-based practice. Work patterns and scheduling dynamics—high ratio of part-time nurses coupled with a multitude of shift lengths and various shift start times—are causing major impediments to continuity of care, the bedrock of relationship-based practice.

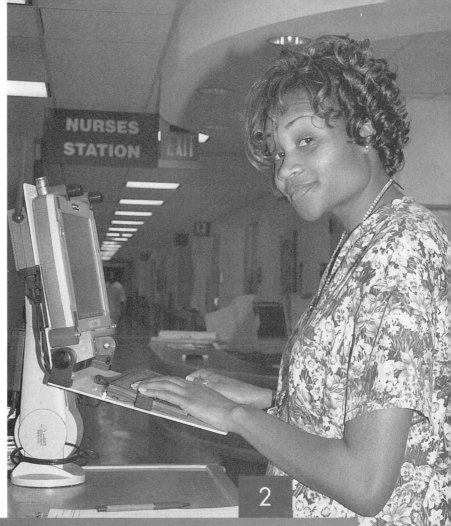

The Twenties, Thirties, Forties, Fifties and Sixties

2

What has happened to nursing since the twenties that paints such a bleak picture? An oversupply of nurses resulted in underemployment in the twenties and yet by the fifties and sixties there were severe shortages, reflecting profound changes in society. From a private practice conducted in patients' homes nursing made the tremendous leap into an enormously *complex* machine and space age health care practice conducted in one of the most complicated institutions known to mankind. To answer the "what happened?" question, we need to look at nursing's reaction to the world events that shaped the course of practice.

The Twenties

In the wake of the First World War, women moved one step closer to liberation by getting the right to vote. The idea of a career appealed to more and more of them, and nursing was viewed as a highly acceptable alternative to teaching. It was just as respectable as a career and still a cut above the other types of employment then available to young women who did not wish to teach. There was no shortage of educational opportunities and the cost was within the means of most middle-class families.

New schools of nursing were springing up everywhere, as newly constructed hospitals, many of them small, private organizations which appreciated the economic advantages of student labor, initiated their own training centers. In 1926 there were 2,155 schools of nursing compared to 1,300 in 1946 [3].

The Thirties

The nurse-power oversupply had kept salaries down, so nurses were poorly prepared to endure the economic hardships of the depression of 1929. Scarce jobs became scarcer as fewer families could afford to feed themselves, let alone hire nurses to care for their sick. The use of hospitals for the care of the ill increased. By the early thirties, nurses were standing in the bread lines and eating in soup kitchens, unable to find enough work to support themselves. During this period, many of them returned to their home hospitals and asked to be allowed to work in exchange for room and board. The hospitals opened their doors to their own graduates and, in exchange for a full week of work, gave them a place to sleep and three meals a day. Although graduate nurses had worked in hospitals prior to this period it was in the capacity of private duty nurses, not as employees of the hospital. As time passed, these nurses were paid a stipend and their role was eventually legitimized by the establishment of job descriptions and regular salaries. At first, however, there was an interesting confusion over the difference there should be in the job description between a senior nursing student and a graduate nurse. After all, talented seniors were head nurses of the wards and in some hospitals even took over when the superintendent of nurses had a day off. Not surprisingly there was concern over the use of salaried graduate nurses in positions which could equally be filled by cheaper student labor. It was under these circumstances that the shift in setting of graduate practice from home to hospital now took place. Never since has the majority of trained practitioners been in private practice.

Since graduate nurses could technically perform all the care a patient required, the case method was used for patient assignments. Individualized patient care was still the focus of their attention; the difference between home care and hospital care was negligible. However, this did mark the first time that graduate nurse practice was subject to the rules and regulations that exist in a bureaucratic institution.

The Forties

Before the nation recovered economically from the effects of the depression, Pearl Harbor was bombed.

The wartime need for trained nurses quickly assumed a priority second only to the need for armed servicemen. Periodically throughout the war serious consideration was given to drafting nurses; the problem, however, was an inadequate supply of trained nurses rather than an unwillingness of those trained to serve. Overnight the oversupply turned into a critical shortage. The federal government heavily subsidized nursing education and the Cadet Corps training programs began producing nurses in unprecedented numbers.

Still, no matter how many were trained, the war required more and more. To relieve the continuing shortage multilevel training programs were developed to teach auxiliary personnel how to perform simple care and technical procedures. In the military services, these programs produced "corpsmen" specially trained for each branch of the armed services at various levels of technical skill. In civilian life two types of auxiliary training programs were developed; a one-year program preparing people to provide technical nursing care, and on-the-job training which prepared people to perform the simplest types of care. The former were called Licensed Practical Nurses, the latter, Nurses' Aides. Nurses' Aide training programs were originally designed and taught by the American Red Cross for housewives who volunteered their time to relieve the extreme nurse shortage in civilian hospitals. These original volunteer aides were often identified by the color of their smocks and so became known as the "grey ladies" or the "pink ladies." By the end of World War II, this role had been institutionalized to the extent that most hospitals were providing their own on-the-job training programs for nurse aides. Indeed, for a while, some hospitals had two aide job descriptions: one for paid aides and one for unpaid, or volunteer aides. Simultaneously the Licensed Practical Nurses found a permanent place in the hospital hierarchy.

Meanwhile, wartime acquisition of medical knowledge and technological developments grew tremendously, resulting in enormous increases in the size and complexity of hospitals. New developments and techniques acquired on the battlefield were brought back to the home front as quickly as the knowledge could be acquired and the nature of care given in hospitals changed beyond recognition, especially in the fragmentation of complex procedures.

Toward the end of the war, as projections were being made for peacetime needs, nursing leaders feared that nursing would once again suffer the economic hardships experienced before the war. The phenomenal number of cadet nurses returning to the United States, coupled with the unprecedented preparation of auxiliary workers trained in many of the simpler aspects of hospital care was expected to drive salaries down to prewar levels. In the event, of course, this did not happen. Instead, the overwhelming shortage of nurses persisted and was a major concern to providers of health care for the next twenty years.

The Fifties

Much of the nursing research of the fifties was devoted to developing delivery systems for acute care settings that would facilitate the use of auxiliary workers (LPN's and NA's) in providing direct nursing care under the supervision of registered nurses. In 1948, Esther Lucille Brown [4] exhorted the profession to develop ways to use the people already trained and pleaded for the establishment of nursing services that were differentiated but integrated. The resulting development projects and research efforts culminated in the design of team nursing.

The postwar building boom experienced throughout the country was especially great in the hospital industry. To make sure that adequate beds were available the federal government passed the Hill-Burton Act to furnish new buildings. Hospitals were erected in communities that had previously had none and wings were added to existing buildings. During these years, health manpower education and training programs could not begin to keep up with the increase in hospital beds. Ever greater pressures were exerted on the nursing profession to prepare more and more registered nurses. Many hospitals had whole wings or floors that were unoccupied because of insufficient staff.

Throughout the United States and Canada, the late fifties and the sixties were years of trouble and frustration for staff nurses and nurse administrators. The postwar shortage of nurses became a chronic problem that threatened to hold back the unprecedented growth in medicine and hospitals. The shortages were of nurses, not dollars. Recruitment competition was fierce. Attractions such as low-cost housing, tuition-free courses, and free holiday weekends became standard incentives. One hospital located in the heart of "automobile city" offered graduates options on cars bearing the same name as the hospital. The recruitment ads in journals looked like marriage broker ads.

The problem of the chronic undersupply of nurses coupled with the unprecedented growth in hospital beds was compounded by: 1) the ever increasing complexity of new technological procedures and 2) a persistently high turnover of nurses.

> A recent study of some 325 hospitals showed that about 20 percent of the positions for professional nurses were vacant, as were 18 percent of the positions for practical nurses. In New York City, over half of the positions for professional nurses in the public hospitals were unfilled in 1961. In all hospitals in Los Angeles, private as well as public, 25 to 30 percent of the positions for professional staff nurses are reported as unfilled. In a recent survey of all general hospitals in the State of Massachusetts, it was found that 20 percent of the positions for professional staff nurses were not filled [5].

These vacancies were in existing financed positions, not wishful dreams! The modern nurses of the sixties had become mobile. It seemed as though suddenly they had discovered that they could move to any corner of the US and find a nursing job. The shortage was nationwide. A nurse employed in a hospital with short staffing could resign, move to another part of the country, and count on being employed by another hospital with an equally severe problem; only the scenery was different. The number of nurses who did just this caused a turnover rate that created appalling staffing problems for nurse managers. These chronic shortages and high turnover rates among nurses led in turn to an increased reliance on the more stable caregivers in nursing's workforce: aides, orderlies and licensed practical nurses.

> This pragmatic solution to the problem of shortages has produced an alarming dilution of the quality of services. In some hospitals the use of auxiliary workers has reached such extreme proportions that nursing aides give as much as 80% of the direct nursing services [6].

The need to utilize these auxiliary workers was undeniable; the challenge to nursing was to create an organization for them at the station level that would facilitate their maximal utilization under the control and supervision of registered nurses.

During the fifties, the concept of team nursing in its present sense developed and swept the country. By the mid-sixties, if a hospital was not using this model, its nursing care was considered inferior by the nursing community. In implementing team nursing, hospitals divided stations of any size into two teams, each to be directed by a registered nurse called a "team leader," on two, if not all three, shifts. The team leader supervised and coordinated all the nursing care activities performed by team members who were usually LPNs, and Nurses' Aides, and sometimes RNs. For example, the team leader was responsible for seeing to it that everything ordered for all the patients on her team was administered in a timely fashion. In addition to these "foreman" activities, the team leader was responsible for providing professional direction in the care rendered by the less prepared team members.

To nurse administrators obsessed with the problems of nurse shortages this seemed an ideal way to utilize RN's maximally; to hospital administrators, team nursing appeared a way to hold down professional salary costs by using cheaper labor, and, to at least some nurses, it created a role that enabled them to be one step removed from what was perceived as the menial work of bedside nursing. *Most* nurses really lamented being removed from bedside care, but to be against team nursing in the sixties was like being opposed to moon walks in the seventies.

The Sixties

By the mid-sixties, the roar of dissatisfaction had reached a crescendo. Patients were dissatisfied with hospital care, physicians were dissatisfied with nursing, and nurses were dissatisfied with themselves and everyone else. The public used the popular press as a forum to express its unhappiness with hospital care. Nurses expressed theirs by continuing to switch hospitals, by leaving hospital nursing, and by leaving nursing altogether with alarming frequency. In large hospitals, it was not unheard of to run five hundred nurses through orientation programs in one year! During the middle sixties this author studied some characteristics of the nursing staff at the University of Minnesota Hospitals and found the average length of time a new graduate stayed on the job was seven months. In some positions there was 1300% turnover-three nurses in one position in one year. Kramer's work accurately describes the dimensions of the problem [7].

Nurse administrators faced two major problems: 1) patients were receiving fragmented, depersonalized and discontinuous care, and 2) nurses were discouraged and frustrated with their jobs. Unfortunately, the two problems were, and often still are, treated as one. The belief seems to be that if the profession of nursing is strong and healthy (and nurses are happy) then patients will naturally receive better nursing care. This may or may not be true. The juxtaposition of the two problems leads to a concentration of all energy and attention on solving nurses' problems and not enough on the problems of poor patient care.

Within nursing the focus was now on the concept of professionalism. Efforts to define the word "professional" came to center on a differentiation based on the educational preparation of practitioners. Two-year community college-based schools of nursing began replacing the hospital diploma programs, enabling a clearer delineation of levels of preparation. The American Nurses Association position paper of 1965 used the word "professional" to describe the practice of nurses who had been graduated from baccalaureate programs and "technical" to describe the practice of a graduate of an associate degree or diploma program [8]. An unfortunate result of the position paper has been the obscuring of the basic meaning of the word "professional."

15

Meanwhile, efforts were being made to isolate the "unique" body of knowledge that would "belong" to nursing and to nursing only. Frequent curriculum revisions became the rule rather than the exception and as the clinical component of nursing was de-emphasized, confusion and ambiguity concerning its boundaries inevitably grew. Nurse educators and administrators disagreed widely about the appropriate content of nurse education programs. Today the divergence in expectations of new graduates between educators and administrators is so wide many fear the chasm that exists can never be bridged.

At the graduate level nursing education swung, within a period of a very few years, from functional (education or administration) to clinical (medical/surgical, maternal-child, pediatric, and psychiatric nursing, etc.). Clinical specialists prepared at the master's level arrived in hospitals and nurse administrators began the still unfinished search for an appropriate job description that would ensure the most effective utilization of this most highly educated clinical nurse.

Because the problems within nursing and the problem in taking care of hospitalized sick people were often seen as one and the same, the ferment in nursing education had a powerful effect on nursing service. Some nurse administrators, in an attempt to implement the position paper of the American Nurses Association, tried to reserve the team leader role for graduate nurses with "BSN" after their names. The "professional nurse" was seen as the RN with a baccalaureate education who was prepared to develop a comprehensive care plan "based on nursing process" (sic). The morale problems created when someone without a bachelor's degree was hired as a team leader were very depressing. The efforts to define professional practice on the basis of educational credentials in the sixties left a legacy of second-class citizenship issues in the seventies that promise to remain with us for many decades to come.

Nurse administrators, mindful of the efforts to identify the unique body of knowledge that is nursing's alone, and in an effort to solve the manpower shortage problem, began to analyze the non-nursing activities being undertaken by nurses. Activities that were clearly non-nursing tasks were freely given away to other departments. So, in the sixties, nurses stopped washing beds of discharged patients, and housekeeping departments began cleaning all kinds of substances, even material produced by the human body. Pharmacy departments began automatic replacement programs for floor stocks of medications, dietary departments began passing nourishment and drinking water, and laboratory services began doing venipunctures. New tasks were no longer delegated to nurses just because physicians were no longer interested in performing them. Requests for nurses to accept delegated medical tasks were now subject to new scrutiny by nursing administration and *if* certain criteria were not met, the tasks did not become nursing responsibilities. If a "DMT" did not seem to "belong" to the "unique" field of nursing, responsibility for its performance was not accepted by the nursing department. (However, by the *time* a director of nursing received the request to train floor nurses to perform a new task, such as taking central venous pressures, she usually discovered, to her chagrin, that ICU nurses had been doing it for Dr. So-and-so for the past six months.) Since there was no consensus about the content of the unique field of nursing, the decision about whether or not to take on a new DMT was usually decided in the negative because of workload impact. When the starting of IV's was no longer an intern's job, special IV teams were developed because nursing could not take on that additional workload: As IPPB treatments became popular, new departments of inhalation/respiratory therapy developed. Indeed, many hospitals went so far as to train lay people to administer medications to patients in an effort to relieve the workload of the registered nurses. The transference of "non-nursing" tasks to other departments, and the development of special teams to perform therapies too time-consuming for floor nurses were some of the means used to offset the excessive demands being placed on the inadequate supply of nursing resources. The establishment of unit management departments to relieve nurses of paperwork was another avenue vigorously pursued by hospital and nursing administrators in the latter half of the 1960s to "free the nurse to nurse."

Nurses thus "freed," however, were still so harried and harassed trying to cope with the army of caregivers that arrived on the station each day, that patients were frequently heard apologizing before they requested an essential service from the rushed nurses: "I know you're busy but…" The coordination of the army was difficult since nurses had no real authority over them; however, when something went wrong it was easy to know whom to blame since the nurse was the one with the cap on. (Significantly by 1968 staff nurses and nurse administrators in many hospitals were locked in battle over the issue of whether or not the wearing of caps was mandatory.)

By the late sixties, the majority of clinical bedside care was being given by NAs and LPNs, supervised by RNs who also performed some of the more complex tasks, such as adding medications to the IVs. Hordes of technicians requiring information and coordination arrived daily on the station at their department's convenience to perform technical procedures on patients. As caps and uniforms ceased to identify who was performing which services and functions, patients became thoroughly confused about who was doing what for them. Although nurses were spending more and more time in communication-related activities it became less and less realistic to expect a team leader to know the names and diagnoses of the patients on her team. It is not unfair to say that patients did not know which caregivers were nurses, and nurses did not know who their patients were or why they were in the hospital.

Solutions of the Sixties

Two of the most popular solutions put forth during the sixties were unit management, in which non-nurses managed many stations, and more nurses. Since patients' loudest complaints were about dehumanized care, and nurses' loudest complaints were about insufficient help and too much paperwork, nurse administrators concentrated on getting more nurses and reducing the clerical chores. The assumption was that this would result in better patient care, or happy nurses equal happy patients! By 1967, the University of Minnesota Hospitals were ready to give serious consideration to developing a department of unit management. This author and other nurses visited hospitals in various states to study their experiences before launching such a department ourselves.

Accompanying us on these trips was an associate hospital administrator. At each hospital he would ask his counterpart two questions: "How much does unit management cost in new salary dollars?" and "What effect has it had on patient care?" We were dismayed when the answer to the first question was, in some cases, as much as $500,000 in new salaries with no commensurate reduction in the nursing budget. But the answer to the second question was even more discouraging. The few hospitals that had conducted before-and-after studies of how nursing time was utilized found that there was little or no significant change in the amount of time devoted to direct patient care. I had great difficulty understanding and accepting this fact. In hospitals where virtually all the paperwork was handled by non-nurses, not to mention such functions as supply-ordering, equipment and environmental maintenance, nurses were still not spending more time with patients; I began to wonder if it was a matter of being *able* or being *willing*.

As I began analyzing this question I searched the literature to develop a better understanding of the relationship between staffing and the quality of care. An Investigation of the Relation between Nursing Activity and Patient Welfare, a study done by Myrtle Kitchell Aydelotte at the University of Iowa, produced some startling results [9]. And numbers of station personnel varied staffing. Data were collected before and after each staffing change to determine what effect different patterns had on the quantity and quality of the care the patients received. The most startling finding (consistent with the others, but more dramatic) was the design whereby professional staff assigned to a patient care unit was increased by sixty percent. Measurements of the amount of time the greatly expanded staff spent with patients were made and *there was no significant increase!* The sixty percent more time available was spent on the station, but *not in the patients' rooms!* It was spent at the desk, in the "john," at coffee, charting, talking to house staff, etc. Anywhere, but *not in the patients' rooms!*

Thus, it seemed that neither of the two popular solutions to the problems of hospital nursing services was really effective; neither unit management nor more nurses necessarily had the desired effect of increasing the amount of time nurses spent caring for patients or of ensuring greater patient satisfaction with that care. The solutions did create more time but it was not being spent at the bedside.

And so the question became: Was the nurse shortage one of actual numbers of nurses or was it a problem in the ways nurses were being utilized? Once that question began receiving serious attention, energy formerly directed at recruitment, turnover, scheduling, etc., began being applied to an analysis of what nurses actually did and how they did it.

At the University of Minnesota, staff nurses and leaders working on the unit management project station (by now called "Project 32," so named because the pilot station was number 32), focused attention on that question and decided that before any major modification in hospital structure, such as a unit management department, was undertaken, efforts should be made to streamline the delivery of nursing service. The intent was to ensure appropriate utilization of nurses under unit management while avoiding the expensive pitfalls in the systems used by other hospitals.

It should be noted that this attention was still focused on ways to improve the implementation of *team* nursing. There was a strong feeling that more effective team nursing (following the book's directions more exactly) would certainly result in better planned, more coordinated and more comprehensive patient care.

In an effort to discover just how team nursing had been incorrectly implemented, three major problem areas were identified and concentrated upon: 1) the fragmentation of care; 2) complex channels of communication; and 3) shared responsibility and lack of accountability. Efforts to solve these problems by improving the implementation of team nursing were as unsuccessful in this instance as they had been in all others. However, in this case they led to the establishment of an alternative organization which eventually came to be called Primary Nursing. Its design was a direct reaction to the inability of the team system to deliver nursing care that was coordinated, individualized, and comprehensive; instead of fragmented care, the case method is used; instead of complex channels of communication, simple direct patterns are used; instead of shared responsibility, individual responsibility is clearly allocated.

Problems of Team Nursing

Fragmentation of Care

Team nursing was supposed to facilitate effective utilization of auxiliary workers (LPN's and NA's) under the direct supervision of registered nurses. To accomplish this tasks were *divided up into the simplest components*, and then graded and matched to the skill levels of these workers. Thus, Nurses' Aides took all the temperatures; LPN's took all the blood pressures; Registered Nurses passed all the medications. From the patient's point of view, this form of work allocation required relating to at least three and usually many more members of the staff on each of the three daily shifts. When work assignments are divided in this way the reward and punishment structure that motivates individuals centers primarily on their timely completion. Thus, the aide who is taking the eleven o'clock temperatures is in a hurry to complete them so she can help pass lunch trays that arrive at 11:20. Similarly, the registered nurse passing the 9:00 a.m. medications is in a hurry to get them out on time otherwise "meds will be late" and the ugly question of whether or not there was an "error" due to lateness may have to be addressed. Patients requesting personal care of this aide or RN are soon made to realize that their care needs are *interrupting* important work assignments. The underlying assumption here seems to be that if all of the different bits of care are administered on time (which is, in any case, obviously not always possible) patients will have received good, comprehensive care. The fundamental flaws in this assumption demand close scrutiny.

Complex Channels of Communication

The fragmentation of care that resulted from a task-based method of work assignment led to the second problem of complex communication channels. As we examined further what nurses did and how they did it at our hospital, we found inordinate amounts of time being spent in activities related to communication. Despite this, however, I remained uneasy about the amount of knowledge nursing staff members actually had about their patients. As the communication problem was studied, we found highly complex patterns in use in shift reports. The following example depicts the magnitude of the problem:

On one busy surgical station, the head nurse often arrived a half hour early (to get a head start) and received the morning report from the night nurse. She then relayed the report to the team leaders who later gave it to team members. Patient condition information was thus sifted through three minds and subjective evaluations before it became data to be used by those giving direct care to the patients. At the end of the shift, the process was reversed; team members would tell their team leader what had been going

19

on all day with their patients, the team leader would report to the head nurse who would report to the evening charge nurse who would report to the evening team leaders who would eventually give the patient condition report to the evening team members.

Another example of the complexity of the communication channels was seen in an examination of the typical reactions to a change in the patient's condition. The team member who observed the condition change in the patient reported it to the team leader (who might or might not verify it personally). The team leader would then tell the head nurse, who called the physician; he would tell the head nurse what actions to take, which she would pass on to the team leader who would then tell the team member taking care of the patient what to do about it. In identifying this elaborate hierarchy of information channels in team nursing it was obvious to many of us that despite all of these time-consuming reporting and communication mechanisms, the people actually administering the care often did so *with little or no knowledge either of the patient or the problem* for which he was being treated, As one Primary Nurse said:

> *I did team nursing before where one person took the vitals, another person passed the meds and you really didn't get to know your patients and what was going on with them and you were lucky if at the end of the day you had, enough information to pass on to the next shift and you really didn't have the full and complete picture but just bits and pieces of it.*

Shared Responsibility and Lack of Accountability

The third difficulty which we identified and tried to correct in team nursing was eventually seen as having three interrelated aspects: 1) the problem of *shared responsibility*; 2) the problem of *the blank space under the words "nursing care plan;"* and 3) the problem of *the role of the team leader*.

The problem of shared responsibility can be looked at both as it applied to completing the tasks of care and as it applied to care plans. The team leader assigned all the tasks, but she was also responsible for making sure that everything was done on time. So, if a team member forgot to perform a certain procedure when it was due, she could always say to the team leader, "You forgot to remind me." This sharing of responsibility for performing care tasks meant that if something was not done, no one person could be blamed. Shared responsibility equals no responsibility.

Care plans have always created problems, but especially so in team nursing. In the first place, a care plan is supposed to be the result of a care conference. Everybody on the team is supposed to contribute to its development. (The clear implication was that no one member of the team was smart enough to develop a plan by herself.) Since there are only five days a week when conferences can be scheduled, five care plans would be the most that could be generated, This, coupled with a high turnover of patients, always made it impossible to achieve the dream of an up-to-date care plan for each patient. But no team leader need feel too bad about not having a full complement of care plans because when she went off duty, another nurse with the same imprecise degree of responsibility assumed the same role with the same limitations. Everybody was responsible for all patients, so no one was responsible for any one patient.

The blank space under the words "nursing care plan" is a problem that has consumed the time, attention and energy of large segments of nursing's leadership for the past thirty years. They might well have asked who dreamed up the idea in the first place because it certainly does not derive from a need consciously identified by staff nurses.

No other single issue, thought, technique, problem, or phenomenon in nursing has received as much attention, has been as much written about, taught, talked about, worked at, read about and cried over, with so little success. No other issue in nursing has caused so much guilt-energy to be misspent. Yet, no other piece of paper in the hospital system is as devoid of information as that entitled "nursing care plan" unless Joint Commission is coming or students have recently worked on the floor.

Why? How do new graduates learn to give adequate care so quickly without using the basic tool upon which their educational process was based? Anyone who has spent any amount of time in nursing service at any level in any reasonably good hospital knows that, in fact, top-drawer nursing care can be delivered without nursing care plans. Nursing care plans present one of the most stubborn problems faced by modern nursing and it seems that no matter what is said, done or written about them, their use still remains a serious problem. Why has it been so intractable?

First of all, I do not believe nurses avoid writing care plans because they do not care about the continuity of nursing care, nor do I believe that lack of time is the real reason for the blankness of that piece of paper. Anyone who has been in nursing service for any length of time knows that there are many reasons and many excuses given as to why: the plans are not consistently completed. Among the most popular of these are:

- Not enough staff.
- They take too long.
- Nobody reads them.
- They get outdated too soon.
- Nursing care plans are not a part of the permanent record and, therefore, not important.
- Nursing care plans are a part of the permanent record and, therefore, of limited value as a communication tool.
- The head nurse doesn't pay any attention to them, so why should I bother?
- The head nurse doesn't care if they're done or not.
- We give good care without them.

Of all these reasons/excuses, inadequate time is the most difficult to refute and, therefore, the one most frequently used. To be sure, nurses never have enough time to give the kind of care they would like to give. However, it is also true that nursing care plans are the easiest responsibility to neglect since the system offers no immediate sanctions for failing to complete them.

With the shared responsibility and lack of accountability inherent in team nursing, everyone can feel guilty about the absence of care plans, as witness the great variety of excuses, but no one really has to do anything about them. One Primary Nurse commented:

I was finding that in team nursing a lot of things were getting missed and that a lot of people weren't caring about these things getting missed. There were a few people who really cared but they knew it couldn't make a difference when there were so many that didn't care. Here it seems like everyone really cares about their patients. In

21

team nursing they could just pass the buck. Things could just be moving along from one shift to the next but here everyone is really responsible and here everyone is so happy.

The third aspect of the problem of shared responsibility is the role of the team leader. It is most easily illustrated by the challenge a head nurse faces in the orientation of a new graduate. The latter usually has to be taught how to be an effective team leader as quickly as possible so that the staff nurse vacancy which has existed for some time can be filled as quickly as possible. Anxious to practice her newly acquired nursing skills in her first real nursing job, she may or may not have had some experience as a team leader during her student experience. At any rate, the pressure is on both of them to groom her for the role as quickly as possible.

The first thing the new graduate has to learn is how to listen to and retain great masses of verbally transmitted data at morning report. The information may be needed at any time during the coming shift, or not at all, but she must still be prepared to retrieve any of it from her brain cells at a moment's notice. The data may be clinical, social, factual and/or impressionistic and be about a large number of patients. Others can forget; the team leader cannot.

Next, our new graduate must be taught how to make out daily assignments. She first must learn the job description limitations that exist for LPNs and Aides, and then she must learn the real limitations who can actually do what and how much help various team members will require. In learning who should take care of which patients the new graduate will be taught not to assign herself to any patients if she can possibly avoid it. In this way she will be free to help everyone and make sure that all the work is being accomplished according to schedule. However, if staffing is very low, she learns that she may have to assign herself to a few patients. If so, she is instructed to take those who are least seriously ill so she can be as free as possible to supervise the work of the other team members. Thus, the RN, who is the ranking professional on the team, is steered toward the care of those who need least help.

Next, there is "rounds with a purpose." When I left team nursing there were still hot discussions on whether or not rounds could be incorporated with the administration of medication, or if separate rounds "with a purpose" were not more beneficial. I never really did understand the "purpose" but I am sure there was one.

The new graduate has to learn how to schedule staggered coffee breaks for the team members and to schedule lunch periods so the staff gets to eat without jeopardizing lunch tray deliveries. Afternoon cleaning chores also have to be assigned along with special procedures and new admissions.

Finally, the team leader has to learn how to check with the team members at the end of the shift to find out how all the patients have fared that day, so she can give a comprehensive report to the evening team leader. When the new graduate is able to accomplish all that and get everyone off duty by 3:30 p.m. (because the hospital surely does not want to pay overtime), then the head nurse can say, "Wow, she's good!" It is entirely possible that neither she nor, for that matter, the new graduate, has had an opportunity to assess in any meaningful way the quality of clinical judgment our new team leader brings to the bedside.

It is fair to say that team nursing is a delivery system for nursing that requires enormous amounts of time to be spent in communication, but where it is not expected that nurses will know the diagnosis of a patient. It is a system that takes the individual with the highest license to care for the sick and tells that person to care for no sick people except the least seriously ill. It is a system in which what is assigned is not patient care, but tasks. The assumption is that if all of these are done on time, especially morning baths, patients are getting good care.

In 1964, during the heyday of team nursing, the author was asked by her director of nursing to study one particular station at a major teaching hospital where the head nurse was having problems managing patient care. The method used to study the station was described in the United States Public Health Service booklet entitled "How to study Activities in a Patient Unit" [10]. The following excerpts from that report depict typical problems experienced with team nursing.

> Presently, each team member has responsibility for the care of seventeen to eighteen patients. This care is given by three to five team members who have varying levels of skills and education. With a team this large, the activities team leaders have time for are assigning patients to team members, administering medication, doing treatments on patients assigned to nurse aides, charting, giving and receiving verbal communication about patients, and periodically checking patients' conditions. They do not usually have time to accompany doctors on rounds, to teach patients about pre- or postoperative care, to conduct team conferences, or to acquire an understanding of the psycho social aspects of the patients' illnesses.

> …team leaders need an opportunity to acquire information about, and understanding of, the medical care plan. They should be able to accompany doctors on rounds and become familiar with the medical plan. This is essential if nursing care is to be coordinated with the patient's medical treatment…the nursing staff is often caring for patient without current information about the medical plan.

> This activity analysis showed team leaders spending less than half their time with patients while the other half was spent communicating about patient care and handling equipment and supplies [11].

The first attempt to solve these three problems focused on improvements in the implementation of team nursing, with the goal of providing humane, individualized, comprehensive and continuous nursing care. Team leaders on the day shift were asked to take one or two patients for whom each of them would be the "principal responsible nurse." During this phase of implementation, the innovation was actually called PRN nursing. Without relinquishing any of their team leadership responsibilities, they tried to develop comprehensive care plans that would be operative 24 hours a day, seven days a week for one or two selected patients. Within a short period of time, it became apparent that the supervisory aspects of their team leader roles were all consuming; RNs had no time or energy left to concentrate on the needs of a particular patient or two. That kind of concentration would only have had the effect of shortchanging all the other patients as well as reducing the team leader's availability to the team members. After a couple of months it became apparent that if staff nurses were going to be effective in providing nursing care to sick people, then their use as foremen or supervisors over large numbers of patients had to cease.

The decision to try assigning twenty-four-hour-a-day responsibility to all staff nurses, each one having a small case load and having her care decisions be in effect even when she was not on duty seemed a worthwhile way to try to accomplish the patient care goals identified above. Within two weeks, the staff's enthusiasm had infected all of us working on "Project 32." The system was then dubbed" Primary Nursing and the revolution was underway!

Addendum to Chapter Two

My understanding of the history of nursing from the twenties to the sixties covered in Chapter Two hasn't changed. There followed a decade of change and transformation for nursing practice. Led by changes in practice settings, rather than educational institutions, it is a decade marked by pioneers and transformational leaders. I believe the unfreezing of hospital-based nursing began with the love affair with unit management. The late sixties was marked by strenuous efforts to relieve bedside nurses of the non-nursing management activities that inevitably become part of nursing's responsibilities in hospitals. When it became clear from research that unit management, in and of itself, made no impact on bedside practice, there were efforts to change care delivery and the way nursing departments were managed. (University of Iowa study)

In the late sixties, as we were developing Primary Nursing at the University of Minnesota Hospitals, three other nurse leaders in four separate venues simultaneously studied the idea of decentralization. It was only a few years ago, during a conversation at a national conference, that this convergence of an idea surfaced. During the late sixties, Joyce Clifford was teaching in a Master's Program in Nursing Administration at the University of Indiana. She taught her students about the theory of decentralization and its potential impact on the way nursing departments operated. Simultaneously, Janet Kraegle, Virginia Mousseau, et al. were implementing decentralized organization of supplies and care-support materials, revising the physical characteristics of a unit to achieve a point-of-use supply-distribution system. At the same time, Rosamunde Gabrielson implemented a decentralized administrative structure at Good Samaritan Hospital in Phoenix, Arizona. Decentralization was clearly an idea whose time had come.

Pioneers

Throughout the seventies, I continued to explore the principles and implementation of the care delivery system as they affected management and administration. The first published explanation of Primary Nursing was an article in 1970 in a relatively obscure nursing journal, *Nursing Forum*. [Manthey, M., et al. (1970). Primary nursing. *Nursing Forum*. IX.1:65] The first public explanation took place in a seminar at the University of Minnesota in 1971. Interest in the concept steadily grew, and pioneering nurse executives throughout the United States opened their organizations to this development. Actually, the pioneers existed at many levels. Sometimes a nurse manager would hear about the idea, and bring it to her unit, occasionally the only one to make the changes in that hospital. I experience the privilege of meeting them today at conferences and having them share their early experience of Primary Nursing with me.

I cannot recognize all the contributions pioneers made to the concept in the seventies. Two people, however, merit mention in this regard. June Werner, of Evanston and Joyce Clifford, of Boston Beth Israel implemented the Primary Nursing concept with such integrity to the concept that the level of professional practice achieved during their tenure stands like an eternal flame, ever reminding us of the importance of leadership.

Financial Consultants Drive Practice Changes

For the last twenty years, financial and technological changes in society have continued to drive practice changes. Financial consultants introduced cost savings spread over clinical practice in surprising and unwelcome ways. For example, role differentiation was obliterated and generic categories of health care workers were created. Skill-mix changes were introduced to reduce salary costs. Work-redesign projects did nothing to streamline the work, but were thinly disguised changes in the skill mix designed to save salary dollars by reducing RN numbers. The trend outlined above was euphemistically termed "Patient-Centered Care," an ironic misnomer. The outcome was highly fragmented, task-based nursing that reduced morale and dispirited the most dedicated nurses.

Comparisons of apples and oranges were masked to look "scientific" or at least like "accurate measurements." Talented nurse executives who could not accept the consultants' recommendations and still feel confident that nursing care was delivered competently left of their own accord or were fired. The extraordinary turnover of nurse executives in the nineties destabilized nursing departments, already assaulted by the development of service-line management. This marketplace-derived organizational structure eliminated discipline-specific departments, including nursing, by giving authority over staffing budgets to individuals with responsibility for specific product line, such as cardiovascular, otho/neuro, etc. This change created new organizational chimneys, while negating the concept of integrated professional clinical services, such as nursing, respiratory therapy, etc.

The nineties left the nursing profession feeling overworked, under appreciated and uninspired. "I love patient care," bedside staff nurses frequently said, "but I hate my job." However, as the 21st century started, nursing began once again to own its destiny. The extreme staffing shortages forced a reidentification with the fundamental values of the profession. And society speaks loudly and clearly of its frustration with today's health care system, demanding humane treatment and identifying nurses as the purveyors of that treatment. It is ironic that as the extreme workload increases and staffing reductions drive nurses out of hospitals, polls show people trust nurses more than any other professional group, including physicians and clergy!

Nursing's Covenant with Society

What I've come to appreciate is how unchanging nursing's covenant with society is, despite the phenomenal changes within society as a whole. As a profession, we have found that changes in the world forced us to alter many aspects of our practice. Medical advances shortened hospitalizations. The Internet gave the public access to vast amounts of information formerly owned by the profession. Health care is now a business. Nursing sought none of these changes.

Nevertheless, we own our response to them. As a profession, nursing has the right and responsibility to decide the amount, degree and kind of nursing care we will deliver to patients within the constraints society and health care systems set. As the profession matures, it is moving away from anger and sadness at the lost opportunities and toward the understanding that within the real-world framework, it is our right and responsibility to deliver our services consistent with our fundamental contract with society.

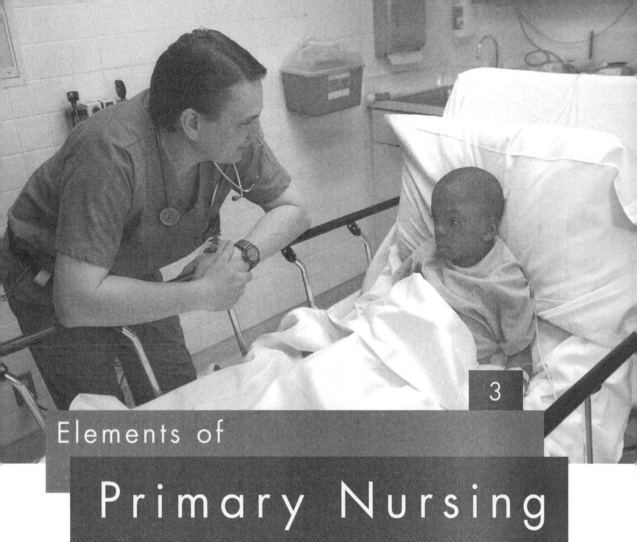

3

Elements of
Primary Nursing

Primary Nursing is a system for delivering nursing service that consists of four design elements: 1) allocation and acceptance of individual responsibility for decision-making to one individual; 2) assignments of daily care by case method; 3) direct person-to-person communication; and 4) one person operationally responsible for the quality of care administered to patients on a unit twenty four hours a day, seven days a week.

The quality of the nursing care thus delivered to patients is determined by the performance of the individuals in the system. Performance is a result of clinical capability, sophistication of judgment, organizational ability and quality of leadership, among other factors.

The quality of nursing service in a Primary Nursing system can be good or bad, comprehensive or incomplete, coordinated or spasmodic, individualized or standardized, creative or routine. Primary Nursing does not define or guarantee the quality of nursing care. As a system, it *facilitates* a very high level of quality by enabling and empowering individuals to perform at their maximum capacity. Whether they do so or not depends on them, not on the system. Thus, Primary Nursing can be in place and the quality of care still be low. It should be pointed out, however, that the quality of care is immediately apparent in this system and those who function at unacceptable levels can be immediately identified and held accountable for their performance. Unacceptable levels of performance can be dealt with appropriately *because* the levels of quality are visible.

Many people have mistakenly equated the concept of a system of care delivery with the concept of quality care. This chapter gives an explanation of the four design elements of the system; role expectations are described in the context of these elements, but whether or not they are met does not determine the presence or absence of Primary Nursing.

Responsibility

The first element, the clear, individualized allocation of responsibility for decision-making about patient care, is the heart of Primary Nursing, the essential difference between it and other systems for delivering nursing care. The Primary Nurse is responsible for deciding how care will be administered to her patients on an around the clock, continuous basis. In functional and case method, decisions are usually made by the head nurse, or charge nurse. In team nursing, decision-making/care planning is the product of a team conference which is led by a team leader, and the care plan is thus the product of a group decision-making process. In Primary Nursing, decisions about a patient's care are made by the bedside nurse who has accepted responsibility for this task.

In addition to deciding how care shall be administered, she personally administers the care whenever possible. This design element recognizes the fact that the person performing an activity is usually the person best able to decide how it should be done. Decentralized decision-making can be defined as putting decision-making authority at the level of action. In hospitals, the action level is the bedside, and the action person, the bedside nurse. The Primary Nurse is both a planner of care and a giver of care. In commenting on the integration of these two functions one staff nurse said

> *I like the freedom I'm allowed. I like the freedom of making my own decisions, deciding what my patients need. I like it because I get more involved with my patients and can learn more about them than I did in team leading. I feel much more satisfied because I have a much better understanding of the patients and all of their needs* [12].

It is essential that this acceptance of responsibility be visible to people within and outside of the delivery system. Thus, the patient, the patient's friends and relatives, the physicians, other nurses and other members of the health team must know the name of the Primary Nurse.

There are three major areas of concentration required in the exercise of this responsibility. First of all, the Primary Nurse is responsible for making available the necessary clinical information others need for the intelligent care of her patient in her absence. This means the Primary Nurse must not only be knowledgeable herself but also must be able to recognize what information is essential for the others to have and what is not. The types of areas of significant information are not defined in advance for her; it is up to each nurse to decide this on a patient-by-patient basis. In some cases, it may be the etiology or prognosis of the disease or, in others, the fact that this is a familial disease. In one case it may be the symptoms to watch for, while with another patient it may be important to know that a new form of treatment is being used. In some cases, the Primary Nurse may decide there is no clinical information of significance to be shared with her colleagues; that too is her decision to make.

Second, the Primary Nurse is responsible for deciding how nursing care shall be administered and for making that information available to other nurses in the form of instructions for care. The nursing process is useful in fulfilling this responsibility.

The Primary Nurse collects information using whatever sources are available to her, such as the patient, the chart, the physician, the patient's relatives, etc., and on the basis of the data thus collected develops a preliminary plan of care. Different hospitals provide different tools for use in data collection and writing the plan of care: nursing history forms, Kardex care plans, nursing order sheets, admission guides or whatever. Any of these can be helpful in assisting the nurse in the planning process but their design should in no way restrict the quality or quantity of data collection or the clarity with which the resulting care decisions are made. Decisions about how nursing care should be administered are of a much higher quality when the patient and his family participate in them. Deciding how and when a treatment procedure can best be performed or when hygienic care is most important to a particular patient or what time of day physical therapy is best tolerated can best be made with the full cooperation of a knowledgeable patient. Since the quality of a care decision is vastly superior under these circumstances it is incumbent upon the Primary Nurse to educate her patients so their contributions can be meaningful and useful.

Instructions left by the Primary Nurse are to be followed by others caring for her patients in her absence, unless an alteration is dictated by a change in the patient's condition. When that happens, the nurse's instructions may be modified to deal with the new situation. Otherwise, they are to be followed by the staff members who care for her patient on the other shifts, and her decisions continue in force even after she *is* off duty. Thus, if a Primary Nurse has written a comprehensive plan of instructions for a new diabetic that calls for his injecting an orange for the first time on a shift on which she is not working, the nurse caring for the patient on that shift should supervise, assist or teach the patient how to do the procedure.

A disagreement about how a patient should be treated or instructed must be openly negotiated and resolved but must not be fought out on the battleground of the patient's care plan. Simple differences of opinion should be easily resolved in an adult fashion by the individuals involved; serious conflicts regarding patient care may require the use of conflict resolution skills by the head nurse.

The third area of major responsibility the Primary Nurse has is discharge planning. She is responsible for seeing to it that the patient and his family, if they will be caring for him after he leaves the hospital, have been prepared to do so safely and effectively. If the patient is being transferred to an agency that employs nurses, the Primary Nurse is responsible for transferring the necessary information that will be helpful in facilitating a smooth transition. She should tailor each discharge to each individual patient. For example, nurses in an agency or institution to which the patient is being transferred should be given relevant information in a fashion and degree of detail appropriate to the circumstances. A routine referral form may be all that is needed in one case, while for another patient a supplemental discharge summary letter may be indicated. Quite often certain information will be best supplemented by a personal phone call from the Primary Nurse to the nurse in the nursing home or visiting nurses association.

Occasionally, it may be necessary for arrangements to be made for a nurse to accompany a patient to the other institution. Hospital policies should be constructed to allow for the design of individualized discharge plans.

Daily Assignment: The Case Method

The second design element of Primary Nursing is the case method of assignment. "Case method" simply refers to the way care tasks are assigned on a shift-by-shift basis, namely that one person performs all the care tasks for a particular patient regardless of the skill level of the tasks, within the limits set by that person's job description. The underlying rationale of daily patient assignments determining which care giver shall care for which patient on any given day must be the best possible matching of the needs of the patient with the abilities of the care givers available. Assignments should reflect the use of common sense!

Each person so assigned has responsibility to administer care without frequent reminders. If her job description prohibits the performance of certain required activities, she is still responsible for seeing that someone with the required preparation carries out that task. For example, an LPN who is caring for a patient receiving intravenous I fluids observes the rate of flow, informs an RN when fluids must be added, and sees that this is done at the appropriate time.

Case method assignments are patient centered rather than task centered. Care activities can be grouped during one visit to a patient's room, and the hurry associated with the performance of isolated technical tasks for a large number of patients is eliminated. There is more time to talk with patients, to find out what they need or would like, to learn things about them which may affect care plans or discharge plans. In several situations where, for one reason or another, it was not feasible to implement Primary Nursing in its entirety, switching from team nursing to the case method still represented a considerable improvement. Almost immediately, the hectic, harried atmosphere characteristic of busy team nursing stations became less frantic, with a more measured pace of activities.

Criteria for Patient Assignments

As noted above, the most important criteria for deciding who should give daily care are: 1) the unique needs of each patient, and 2) the skills and particular strengths of the available staff members. Team nursing required the use of the most extensively prepared care giver, the registered nurse, as an overseer of less skilled, less expensive labor. It was not uncommon in such cases for the team leader to assign herself to no patients. In situations where serious staffing deficiencies left no choice the team leader would, illogically, take on an assignment of those patients who were least in need of her advanced skills. In the case method of assignment, nurses and patients are matched according to their needs and abilities, respectively. In this way, the most acutely ill patients are cared for by registered nurses, patients with intermediate degrees of illness are cared for by licensed practical nurses and, if I Nurses' Aides are used to give direct care, it is to the least acutely ill patients.

Geography, or the location of patients' rooms in relation to each other should have little, if any, effect on assignment decisions. Admittedly, the head nurse is challenged with needing a better knowledge of her staff's abilities in order to match these optimally to patients' needs, whereas geographically based assignments are much easier, but it is the head nurse's job to know her staff. Assignments based on patient room locations would make sense only if the top priority were to reduce the number of steps the staff nurses have to take on a given shift. However, while the assignment of patient rooms next to each other would seem to save walking time the fact is that the clustering of care activities for each patient made possible by the case method reduces the number of steps and the amount of time spent walking from one patient's room to another most effectively.

However, zones, districts or modules are enjoying a certain amount of popularity as determinants of the assignment process, despite the fact that they ultimately restrict freedom of decision-making and often have a negative impact on unit morale. Such arbitrary rigidity in assigning patients results in an excessive narrowing of a staff member's awareness of all the patients on the station. Geographical assignments result in territorial attention spans. Repeated assignments to care for patients in one geographical area, although intended to enhance continuity of care, often result in the nurse's honestly lacking awareness of the other patients' care needs. This in turn leads to an understandable unwillingness to pitch in and help other nurses or to answer a strange patient's signal light. Geographically grouped assignments can also result in less continuity of assignments on units where patients are frequently transferred from one room to another. Instead of districts, modules or zones, continuity of care is best maintained by having the Primary Nurse administer care personally when she is on duty and by having all other staff members follow her care plan when she is off.

Direct Channels of Communication

The third design element of Primary Nursing was developed to correct the data distortion identified previously as a problem inherent in the communication "pyramid" of team nursing. This element provides for a direct communication channel among the nursing staff members as well as from the nurse to the patient, to the doctor, dietitian, physical therapist, pharmacist, chaplain, etc. This element is simply a flattening of the communication pyramid so that important information is not filtered through middlemen; one care giver communicates directly with another care giver.

Station communications typically center on the shift report as an essential time of information transmission. This design element calls for the care giver on one shift to report directly to her counterpart on the oncoming shift. The actual way in which the shift report is handled is not of particular importance. Tape recorders work fine for some people, and not at all for others. Some groups like walking rounds, while others have staff members moving in and out of the conference room. (Coordination may be a problem. If report begins taking twice as long as before, a change in method should be explored.) Anyone who needs to hear a report should be welcome to attend. If at all possible, charge nurses and all oncoming staff will probably want to listen to the complete report. The only irreducible requirement of this design element is simply that the caregiver on one shift must report to the person who will be caring for her patient on the next shift.

The Primary Nurse is also responsible for initiating communication directly with other members of the health team who either have information she needs or who need information she has. This means that if her patient's IV is to be maintained at 32 drops a minute throughout the time he is in diagnostic radiology, she is responsible for making sure the technician or radiologist caring for the patient during the procedure has this piece of information. Likewise, if there is some aspect of the patient's dietary manage-ment the nurse does not know or does not understand, she is personally responsible for calling the dietitian to get the information. If the nurse wants to know more about the medical treatment plan she is responsible for taking the necessary steps to acquire this information; conversely, if she thus learns of information that she feels the physician should know, she is responsible for communicating it to him. In short, the Primary Nurse is responsible for getting from and giving to any other member of the health team all information which is pertinent to her patient and his needs. (One of the many pleasant corollaries of implementing this aspect of Primary Nursing is that suddenly the rest of the hospital discovers that a station staff consists of many individuals besides the head nurse, each with separate identities and unique contributions to make. The value of this to the nursing staff, and to nurses in general, is obvious.)

The role of a Primary Nurse in communicating with the patient and his family cannot be overemphasized. As she becomes familiar with her patient's personality and his needs for knowledge about his condition, she can perform a very useful function in 1) responding to his requests for further information whenever and however it is appropriate for her to do so, and 2) interpreting his needs for additional knowledge to other members of the health team, especially physicians. Occasionally (particularly when the bureaucracy of the hospital impedes responsiveness to the patient's needs) it will be appropriate for the Primary Nurse to assume an active role as patient advocate.

Responsiveness to the patient's need to know and enlisting his full participation in decision-making is recognized as a strong and positive factor in reducing malpractice suits. Many hospitals view Primary Nursing as an important asset in reducing their potential for law suits resulting from patients' lack of knowledge. The Primary Nurse can be extremely beneficial in interpreting the patient's need for knowledge and making sure physicians and others know how much he needs and wants.

Caregiver as Care Planner

Because in Primary Nursing the power to decide how a patient shall be cared for is allocated to the individual personally responsible for *providing* the majority of that care, the adequacy or inadequacy of the care plan is immediately obvious to the person best qualified to decide how it can be improved. Equally important, because of this integration of the functions of care planning and care giving, the improvement can be implemented without delay.

As a result of the American Nurses Association Position Paper of 1965 many nursing departments attempted to reserve the team leader role for the baccalaureate graduate, the "professional nurse." The thinking was that the professional nurse would be responsible for the process in all respects except the actual implementation of the care plan. The team members, aides, LPNs and RNs with technical preparation, would be the ones to "lay on the hands" and carry out the decisions made by the baccalaureate prepared nurse. The morale problem which inevitably follows from this arrangement is disastrous. It requires in effect that team members undergo a lobotomy each morning when they put their caps on their heads. It requires further that a given team member follow the orders of a team leader who may have had little direct contact with the patient and no firsthand knowledge of his specific care needs, and who may never herself have performed a particular procedure she is prescribing or be as able to judge its adequacy in practice as can the person who actually carries it out. It should be noted too that this arrangement, aside from the morale problem it breeds, has supplied endless ammunition to those physicians who would like nurses relegated to servant status. They seize on the predictable clinical errors to which it gives rise and exhibit them as typical results of nurses' pretensions to decision-making authority, while the benefits that derive from care planning by knowledgeable care providers intelligently and logically assigned remain obscured from their view.

The decision to integrate the roles of care planner and care giver forces a different way of thinking about how to assign nurses with different job descriptions and different skill levels. Reserving the function of care planning to individuals with a particular type of education, regardless of the ability levels of others, is really a form of functional assignment. We think of functional assignments primarily as assigning such care tasks as temperature-taking to an aide, blood pressure readings to an LPN, etc. But assigning the thinking part of nursing, which is what care planning according to the nursing process is, only to individuals with certain letters after their names is part of the same functional approach to work assignments, and suffers from the same unnecessary limitations.

Although thinking and doing are integrated in Primary Nursing, the problem of assigning work according to ability still exists. The approach to this which I advocate is to match patients and nurses according to the predictable needs of patients over time and the known abilities of individuals on the nursing staff. Thus, if a well adjusted, otherwise healthy, middle aged person is admitted to the hospital for an elective appendectomy and the course of hospitalization is expected to be uneventful, a new graduate just learning her role may be the Primary Nurse with or without close supervision by an experienced RN or the head nurse. If the hospital to which the patient is admitted uses selected LPNs as Primary Nurses, one of them could alternatively be assigned to such a patient. However, if the same patient expresses overwhelming fear of anesthesia and is found to be quite hypertensive at the time of his admission, the decision might better be to assign this patient to an experienced registered nurse. Thus, the criteria for the assignment of Primary Nurses include not only a sophisticated judgment of individual nurses' abilities and interests, but also a thorough knowledge of the implications of a patient's medical condition and an early assessment and prediction of his response to hospitalization.

Assuming that level of education does usually have an impact on level of practice and expertise, graduates of baccalaureate programs can generally be expected to perform better with patients

- whose outcomes are not predictable;
- whose care programs are not standardized;

- whose psychological reaction to illness and/or hospitalization are threatening their ability to cope with life.

Graduates of non-baccalaureate programs can generally be expected to give adequate care to patients

- whose care programs are standardized;
- whose outcomes are predictable; and
- whose psychological reaction to hospitalization and/or illness is not threatening his ability to cope with life.

Experience as well as education must be taken into account when assessing an individual nurse's level of expertise in caring for various kinds of patients. Some people learn continuously through life's experiences and grow daily in their understanding and ability to cope with new situations. Others can graduate *summa cum laude* and never learn another thing in the crucible of the real world. Decisions as to who takes care of which patients should reflect sensitivity to and awareness of each individual nurse's ongoing development.

When a station implements Primary Nursing, it is realistic to expect that within a reasonable period of time all registered nurses will be able to function as Primary Nurses with their own caseloads. Of course, defining a reasonable period of time must be done by the individuals in the situation; I personally cannot imagine *any* circumstances in which that period would exceed one year. I believe that all RN's should be able to function as Primary Nurses and, given the time to grow into the role, I believe exceptional licensed practical nurses can too. The system depends on and reflects individual qualities much more than academic degrees. One of the earliest evaluations of it came from a physician who endorsed it but pointed out that "It makes the good nurses look good and the weak nurses stand out like sore thumbs."

A Primary Nurse cares for her own patients on five of the twenty-one shifts into which the work week is usually divided. New graduates, licensed practical nurses, part-time nurses and other Primary Nurses can all be assigned to care for patients whose Primary Nurse is off duty, as Associates to the Primary Nurse. Whatever the individual's job title, or work frequency, she is expected to follow the instructions of the patient's Primary Nurse unless a change in his condition necessitates a modification of them. Therefore, on any given day a Primary Nurse may have under her care her own two, three, or four patients plus (depending on staffing that shift) one, two or three patients of a Primary Nurse who is then off. For her own patients she is continuously developing their care plans; for patients of a Primary Nurse who is off duty, she follows the instructions left on the care plan by the patient's Primary Nurse. One individual may thus be assigned as both Primary and Associate during a single shift.

Role of the Head Nurse

The single most critical role change necessary for the successful implementation of Primary Nursing is that of the head nurse. The skills, behavior and attitudes that make one a successful head nurse in team nursing are different from those necessary for success in Primary Nursing. In team nursing, the successful head nurse is the one who can answer

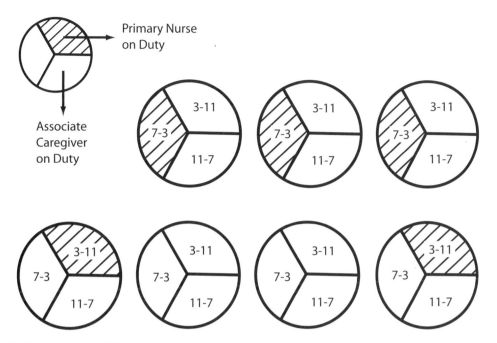

Typical Primary Nurse Shift assignment. In one week the Primary Nurse works five shifts and her associates cover the other sixteen.

everyone's questions and solve a multitude of problems, large and small. The head nurse who knows each doctor's personal preferences, how to get a specimen sent to a lab in Timbuktu, where extra supplies are hidden, and how best to report medication errors is a gem in any system. If in addition to all this she is able to run her floor with a minimum amount of overtime dollars she receives another jewel in her crown. In the team nursing system the hospital world also wants her to know all about each patient's care needs, at least insofar as those needs affect the various services different individuals and departments provide. The physical therapist expects her to know how the patient is doing on bed to chair transfers, the dietitian asks why the patient doesn't eat his sixth meal before bedtime, the physician wants to know whether the patient's abdomen is more or less distended today than it was yesterday and the central supply room wants her to know why this patient needs a scultetus binder instead of one of the new disposable ones. The good head nurse is the font of all of this knowledge and the more accurately and speedily she can answer such questions, the better a head nurse she is.

Rewards for being a good head nurse are powerful in the team nursing system. Most career nurses who were head nurses at some point in their past look at those years with fondness and warm feelings. The job satisfaction from being a "good head nurse" is a unique experience. Physicians, the nursing office, and department heads are powerful reward sources. To be known as a "good head nurse" in those circles is gratifying.

When questioned about the differences between being a head nurse in team nursing and in Primary Nursing one person said,

My sense of satisfaction has changed. In the past it came from knowing it all when dealing with the physicians, but now it comes from seeing the staff feeling good

35

about what they are doing and their development. It makes you feel good seeing them…just as they get satisfaction from seeing their patients do well, I get my satisfaction from seeing them do well.

To make Primary Nursing work, the head nurse has to turn all of those questions over to the staff nurses. Since the Primary Nurse is responsible for direct communication with all members of the health team the head nurse has to learn to refer critical questions to her. In addition to having responsibility for communication, the Primary Nurse actually has greater knowledge of her particular patients. This is often troublesome for head nurses to accept when they have a need to know more than their staff knows. Some head nurses feel insecure when they are known to have less knowledge than their subordinates. In team nursing, it was, indeed, a mark of an ineffectual leader not to know the answers to everyone's questions. In Primary Nursing, however, the head nurse must recognize and respect the superior knowledge the staff has of their own patients. She has to show that respect by declining to answer questions that can best be answered by the care giver, even when she does in fact know the answers.

Everyone is equally respected and there is no power struggle here. Everyone is doing patient care and making decisions and being responsible. Everyone has gone through the pitfalls of making mistakes and knowing that they did something wrong. But they also know that everybody else they work with did that too so they accept each other's mistakes.

I think a lot of it depends on the head nurse. If the head nurse is one who just wants to maintain her power and her control over the floor it's kind of earth-shattering for her to realize that other nurses are going to be able to have the same kind of control…they are going to be able to go to doctors and talk to the doctors about their patient's particular problems and take care of the problems that she used to take care of. A lot of it depends on the head nurse being able to guide the floor and teach the nurses in the change-over [13].

Many head nurses are very uncomfortable with this part of the transition. Once the adjustment to the new communication patterns has been accomplished, the rewards for head nurses begin to focus on nursing practice and the transition will proceed smoothly. They enjoy the satisfaction of watching their staffs' self-image improve, their professional competence become more widely and deeply appreciated and the quality of patient care improve to the extent that patients maintain communication with them even after discharge and, if re-hospitalization is necessary, specifically request a return to the unit of *their* Primary Nurse.

The head nurse role is one of clinical leadership and continuous responsibility for the overall management of patient care. In the area of clinical leadership, the head nurse must be a teacher, the validator of decisions made by her staff, a resource person, and the quality control supervisor for the unit.

As teacher, she is responsible for making sure that every staff nurse has the basic knowledge needed to perform safely on the unit. Whenever deficiencies are noted, the head nurse should either provide the necessary teaching personally or make other arrangements for it. (If teaching occurs without learning, then the head nurse has a personnel management problem.) Beyond basic knowledge, the head nurse ought to set the tone for the staff in striving for growing excellence by pursuing herself the knowledge that will lead to better practice. As a learner she can set a powerful example for the staff by her own continued professional and personal development.

As a validator of clinical decisions made by the staff, the head nurse must acquire the skill either 1) of agreeing with the decision and, hence, validating it, or 2) if she disagrees, of telling the staff member why and suggesting alternative approaches for the staff nurse to use in making a new clinical decision. If at this point the head nurse takes over the decision making authority that rightfully belongs to the Primary Nurse, she will undermine the entire system. Even when a particular nurse wants a decision made for her, the head nurse must be aware of the negative effects of the usurpation of legitimate authority. Decision validation is a new skill required of head nurses in the Primary Nursing System, and time for this kind of learning must be allowed.

As a resource person, the head nurse can fully satisfy the leadership aspects of her role. Because her job is pivotal in the overall operation of the hospital, the head nurse has access to much information that staff nurses do not. Therefore, she is in a better position to know where to get different kinds of help, where particular areas of expertise are to be found and what sources are available to provide different kinds of help. When a staff nurse comes to her with a patient care or patient management problem, a good head nurse will be able to suggest four or five new alternatives for the staff member to explore in solving that particular problem.

Responsibility for the overall quality of nursing care administration on the unit twenty-four hours a day, seven days a week, is the responsibility that most clearly differentiates the head nurse's role from that of her staff. She must be able to evaluate the clinical nursing care decisions made by each of the Primary Nurses to make sure they are adequate, safe and, in any given circumstances, the best possible. To do this, the head nurse has to know the clinical needs and problems of all the patients as well as the strengths and weaknesses of the various members of her staff. She needs to monitor the decisions being made on a regular basis (periodic sampling techniques being quite effective). As performance weaknesses are identified, the head nurse needs to work with the staff nurse to overcome those deficiencies.

A level of supervision has been eliminated from this system, that of the "checker upper for cheaper doers." An implicit assumption is that individual staff members can be trusted to provide the care patients need without frequent reminders. However, if a staff member does not measure up to this assumption it is the head nurse's job either to provide corrective learning experiences or to take appropriate personnel management action.

This responsibility for overall quality of care points to an important consideration of Primary Nursing-station size. During the staff shortages of the 60's, hospital literature reflected a growing concern about the appropriate size of a station. Many articles were written by hospital administrators and hospital architects in favor of quite large stations. (Few articles, if any, have been written by directors of nursing on this subject.) The larger the station, the more economical the staffing was the theme being played. (The expense of salary dollars for head nurses was thus reduced.) As a result, many hospitals expanded station size or built new, larger ones. The question of how many patients one person could care for adequately was not seriously considered as a part of the size equation as put forth by the hospital administrators and architects. In Primary Nursing, however, the importance of this factor cannot be overlooked. When the "checker-uppers" no longer exist and one person is responsible for the management of care on a continuous basis, the question of station size and number of personnel to be supervised becomes paramount. It has been my experience that fifty acute care patients are too many for one head nurse to manage effectively. The clinical knowledge requirement plus the need for familiarity with all the staffs' abilities and deficiencies militate against the implementation of Primary Nursing on excessively large stations.

The Head Nurse as Manager

If a hospital holds the head nurse responsible for the quality of nursing care administered on a twenty-four-hour-a-day, seven-day-a-week basis, authority commensurate with that level of responsibility must also be allocated. Examples of powers which the head nurse must have in order to fulfill her responsibilities include selection of personnel, allocation of resources, evaluation of performance, setting the standards of practice of nursing care, participating in the decisions about how those standards will be accomplished, and the right to terminate those who do not measure up to the standards she sets. If a head nurse is not involved in the selection of personnel, her management authority is eroded. If she does not participate in the evaluation of permanent evening and night staff members, her authority over them does not exist. If she cannot terminate a staff member whose performance is unacceptable, she cannot be held responsible for that nurse's performance. Even though most head nurses have not been prepared to exercise such broad authority, it is vital that they *learn* to do so and *demand the right* to do so. The "who and when" management decisions are of paramount importance to the structuring of a strong role for head nurses. As Jean Barrett wrote as far back as 1949:

> *Good management and congenial working relationships require that no individual should be held responsible for work unless she is granted sufficient authority to prescribe how it shall be done. If she does not have this authority the responsibility for the performance must rest with someone else* [14].

All across the country, head nurses are receiving crash courses in financial management. As cost containment issues capture the minds and hearts of health industry leaders, the issue of controlling dollars spent has become crucial. Head nurses are being taught about salary, expense and revenue budgets. Expenditures excessively over and under the budget require explanations. This new area of responsibility can have a positive effect on strengthening the managerial role of the head nurse. However, unless it is matched by authority to make decisions about revenues and expenditures this new responsibility will become a troublesome burden and liability.

In this author's opinion one of the problems with modern hospitals is that head nurses are held accountable for areas of station operation over which they have no control. All too often this is demonstrated by a head nurse saying something like "I'm sorry, Doctor, I'll see what I can do about that missing lab report," when in point of fact she has no authority over the lab reporting system and, therefore, cannot really do anything about its failure. By apologizing to the physician for every breakdown within the hospital system, head nurses perpetuate the myth that they have control where they actually have none. It would be far healthier for everyone concerned if head nurses were to stop apologizing immediately for those system failures over which they have no control and let those who do experience the consequences of their decision making errors.

The head nurse's role as outlined in this chapter integrates clinical and management components into a single position of strength that includes operational responsibility for competent nursing practice around the clock, every day. Primary Nursing works best where the head nurse is both a good clinician and a good manager. It flourishes in a system where decentralized decision-making is the philosophy of management throughout the department of nursing.

Addendum to Chapter Three

Although changes in the nursing skill mix have always been painful, the impact of RN layoffs in the nineties serendipitously refined Primary Nursing, insuring its survival in the 21st century. When Primary Nursing was first implemented, it was possible for the primary nurse to provide most, if not all, of her own patients' direct care during her tour of duty. I have never had trouble with the use of LPNs in direct care and in fact have always felt there is a strong role in hospital nursing for individuals with that level of technical training. In the beginning, LPNs performed total care for patients whose Primary Nurse was off duty. Nursing assistants performed unit-based support work, and were not assigned to direct patient care.

I always viewed Primary Nursing as a system that could be implemented with the available staff, rather than a system that required special staff, or an all-RN staff. Getting that idea accepted has been an ongoing struggle that was almost lost early on. A research study described an all-RN staffing pattern, using a 1:4 nurse patient ratio. The study was published in a book years before the first edition of *The Practice of Primary Nursing*, and became the reference book of choice, especially since Primary Nursing had only been discussed in journal articles up to that time. Many hospitals used that study to justify substantial increases in their RN ratio, only to have Primary Nursing bonded forever to a certain staffing pattern.

For many, Primary Nursing came to mean RNs do all the care at the bedside. For many, the fundamental principle of decentralized decision-making—the foundation of the system—was never seriously considered: For many, Primary Nursing was simply a staffing and assignment system, with no change in the level of professionalism. The essence of the system is clearly spelled out on page 28, in the description of responsibility:

> *"The first element, the clear, individualized allocation of responsibility for decision-making about patient care, is the heart of Primary Nursing, the essential difference between it and other systems for delivery nursing care."*

The acceptance of responsibility for decision-making must take place within the context of a relationship understood by nurse and patient and by others involved in care throughout the system. Unless the nurse establishes the relationship, it doesn't exist. It is in the act of establishing the responsibility relationship that the nurse *becomes* a professional. Being a professional and understanding the concept of managing a professional practice as a bedside staff nurse in a hospital is the essence of nursing. There are many barriers to accomplishing this; some are logistical, such as scheduling; some are cultural, such as eliminating victim-thinking; and some are personal, such as accepting responsibility for making decisions about the amount, degree and kind of nursing a patient will receive.

As length of stay shortened, ambulatory care increased and the acuity level continued to escalate, while skill mix underwent massive restructuring: It became more difficult for the primary nurse to complete the direct care assignment for her patients. By the mid eighties the "shortage cycle" had reappeared; I was deeply concerned that the demise of the all-RN staff—due to the shortage—would result in the elimination of Primary Nursing. To a certain extent that in fact did happen. Those who equated Primary Nursing with RNs doing total patient care felt they had to give up Primary Nursing. At this time, I began to develop the concept of partnering as a way to employ auxiliary staff, both technical (LPN) and assistive (CNA), at the bedside. We ended up recommending, and continue to do so today, auxiliary personnel work in a relationship with one RN, not assigned to help several. Thus, the concept of pairing or partnering auxiliary staff has mitigated the impact of returning to a lower RN ratio in the skill mix of the staff.

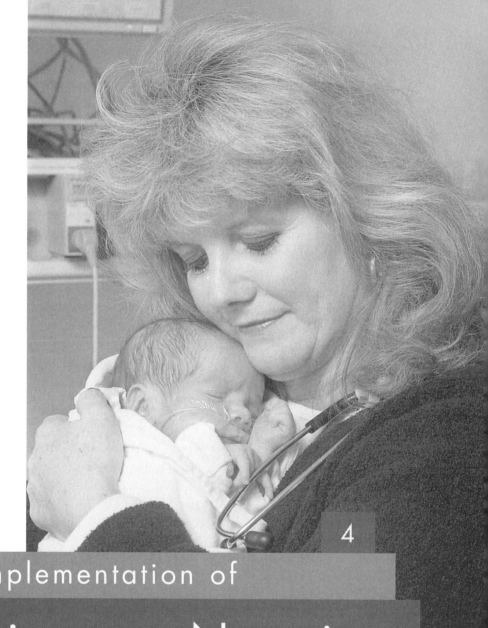

The Implementation of
Primary Nursing

There is no one right way to do Primary Nursing. Each implementation has to be tailored to the setting in which it occurs. A step-by-step cookbook approach is not likely to result in success. The magic formula simply does not exist. In the ten years I have been involved with the system, I have managed or been a consultant to numerous successful implementations and have seen or heard about as many unsuccessful ones. The approach I am recommending in this chapter uses every bit of the real world experience I have had. It is not an easy implementation process, but it is an effective one.

The three factors most instrumental in the successful implementation of Primary Nursing are:

   1. the involvement of station staff members as decision makers;

2. the use of a standard decision-making format;
3. the existence of an effective and supportive management structure.

I have chosen to start by describing the process at the station level because implementation at this level can take place without an institution-wide commitment to Primary Nursing. Later, I will describe the ideal, broader setting in which Primary Nursing flourishes, but readers should not believe that it can *only* exist in ideal institutional settings where the administrative structure is decentralized. Primary Nursing *can* be implemented in any appropriate setting using the process described in this chapter. It is not easy; it requires commitment and courage on the part of the staff. However, the results are the same. A successful implementation results in self-fulfillment of the staff regardless of whether or not the administrative structure supports the system. A successful implementation results in the establishment of relationship bonds among staff members that enable them to provide *each other* with the support not otherwise forthcoming. Risk taking is somewhat riskier, but the rewards are sweeter and the work is just as much fun.

The best way to ensure a successful implementation is to have the right people in key decision-making roles. Since this system is based on a decentralized decision-making model, the key people are those at the level of action, the staff of the nursing station (although it does help a lot if they have the support of their immediate superior). The two basic decisions are:

1. whether or not to implement Primary Nursing, and,
2. how to put the four elements of the system into effect in this particular setting.

These decisions cannot be implemented by management edict. As much as many directors of nursing would like to do just that, the results have usually been disastrous when it has been tried. There are several positive actions a management team can take to facilitate and expedite implementation; but the basic decision of whether and how to implement Primary Nursing belongs to the staff at the station.

At that level, the widest possible participation in decision making is desirable. I personally like to involve anyone who works in the station who wishes to participate, regardless of job category. (I think it far preferable to have a Nurses' Aide or an LPN who is worried about the loss of her own job involved in the planning process instead of outside of it.) The rationale is that since all levels are affected, all levels ought to be able to participate. However, the individuals most affected by the reallocation of responsibility, the staff nurses and the head nurse, *must* be heavily involved in the implementation process. The staff nurses, team leaders and LPN's will have a particularly important role in the implementation process and the head nurse, as formal leader of the group, is the single most important agent in the implementation process. If she is not really in favor of the system and does not support the change, it probably will not work.

Assuming that both the staff and the head nurse are agreed on the decision to implement the system, there remains another preliminary problem which has, in my experience, been the most difficult of all. The staff nurses will usually understand and welcome the difference in their new relationship with the head nurse but of far greater importance and the very foundation of Primary Nursing are their new relationships with each other. Hospital bureaucracies and team nursing neither require nor promote interpersonal relationships among the staff based on mutual trust and respect for one another's total nursing competence; in the absence of individualized accountability they are not particularly important among peers. However, in Primary Nursing the ability of each nurse to deal openly and honestly with others, especially in problem situations, is absolutely essential and must be emphasized from the start.

Old group identifications and territorial attitudes must be changed in the minds of staff members as they are to be changed in the new system. Night shift and day shift, RNs, LPNs and Aides, "old-timers" and "new-comers," etc. are no longer distinctions that have any relevance in Primary Nursing and a conscious effort to replace these with a sense of full and equal membership in the larger professional group must be cultivated. Subgroup identifications die hard, though, and every manifestation of them should be brought out into the open immediately and the healthier, constructive alternative of identification with the total group encouraged.

One subgroup that usually is necessary is a planning group. If the staff is small and communication lines are open and consistently effective, it may be possible to proceed without designating such a group, but stations with a large staff (over twenty people) and the usual communication problems will find that a planning group expedites the process. The selection of the group should take into account the need for representation of all shifts, categories of employees and other special interest groups. It should be small enough to be effective while large enough to represent all segments; usually eight to ten people is the best number. Members of the planning group should serve as two-way communication conduits between the rest of the staff and the group as a whole.

Steps in the Implementation Process

The standard steps of the problem solving or the decision making process apply:

- First, a definition of the problem and making a commitment to explore and evaluate the system;
- second, data collection to ensure a full understanding of the system;
- third, agreement (or as close to it as possible) to implement Primary Nursing;
- fourth, evaluation of the effect of the system change on the delivery of nursing.

The consistent use of this process results in an inherently logical implementation tailored to the needs of the specific situation. While it is not an instant, "magic formula" it can be relied upon to yield results.

Deciding to explore the concept of Primary Nursing is the first actual step of implementation taken by the staff. Discussions leading up to this step usually deal with a consideration of whether or not Primary Nursing is a better system for delivering nursing care than the one currently in use. If the majority of the staff is totally against *even considering* any way of improving patient care there is no point in pursuing the process of implementation. This kind of negative reaction signals the presence of serious morale problems. Most people want to improve; the absence of a desire to do so indicates the need to address other, more fundamental problems before attempting a change in system which presupposes group-wide cooperation. As one nurse summed it up:

43

You really have to feel strongly about it. You really have to want to do it, otherwise as soon as something goes wrong, you can say, "Well, we tried it but it didn't work." You really have to want it. You have to have a strong head nurse who is going to say, "Look, it's going to be tough to do it but it is the best kind of nursing care there is, so we have to do it."

An effective way to start the process is to ask the entire staff to write their answers to the following questions. The written answers are not to be handed in; a verbal exchange of answers is to be encouraged, but not mandated. The more sharing, the better the process, but it must be voluntary.

Registered nurses and licensed practical nurses:

- Why did you decide to study nursing?
- Which parts of your job do you enjoy most?
- Which parts of your job frustrate you most?
- Are your original objectives being met on this job?

Support staff (aides, orderlies, technicians, etc.):

- Why did you accept employment in the nursing department?
- Which parts of your job do you enjoy most?
- Which parts of your job frustrate you most?
- Are your original objectives being met in this job?

Most people enter the nursing field because of a sincere desire to help people. Few enter for the money. Job constraints and frustrations often bury these altruistic motives. It is helpful for the staff to re-experience their earlier motivations, and discussing their answers can be a beneficial process. Again, the more sharing the better and sharing is best when it is voluntary. Some reluctance to talk about this is natural, but refusal to participate at all indicates potentially serious interpersonal relationship problems and warrants the separate attention of the head nurse, independent of the planning sessions.

If a planning group has been appointed, all members should have been in on the verbal discussion as they must have a sense of how the staff reacted. This data provides excellent background information about where people are coming from and where they feel they ought to be headed.

During this preliminary phase, the planning group should address the following questions:

- What are the positive attributes of nursing care on our station?
- In what ways can we improve our nursing care?
- Are most of us satisfied with the results we achieve in patient care?

The answers to these questions which are valid for the group as a whole begin emerging when the personal questions asked are being discussed. Recognition of the positive aspects of care that should be preserved is as important to the success of the change process as is a well developed problem statement. As the strengths and weaknesses of nursing are identified, a statement of the philosophy and the values of nursing for that station can be developed. Whether this is an informal or formal, written or spoken statement does not matter. From a synthesis of these personal assessments the group's level of professional satisfaction can be defined.

Data collection is the second step of the process. (There is not a rigid sequence to these steps; often literature about Primary Nursing appears first and then people begin talking about it.) Articles, tapes, books, personal experiences, etc., are all rich sources of information about Primary Nursing. Conversations and discussions among staff members should be encouraged. Differences of opinion, interpretation, values and meanings are useful opportunities for growth and learning. Individual staff members should be encouraged to think seriously about how this system will affect them personally. A thorough understanding of the system by each individual is important; unthinking acceptance or rejection of someone else's opinion should be pointed out and avoided. The design elements of Primary Nursing are not difficult to comprehend; ignorance due to incomprehension is a poor excuse for passive resistance. The role of staff leadership (both formal and informal) is to encourage openness and honesty. The basis for trust relationships, so helpful after Primary Nursing has been implemented, should be established during this early period of reaction to the system.

Questions quickly surface as information is acquired and digested. To the maximum degree possible, I prefer to see these questions answered on an individual, station-by-station basis. Some questions, indeed, may require a hospital-wide decision for consistency, but I prefer that recommendations even for those come from the staff instead of the management team whenever possible.

The following questions are those which most often have been asked by groups thinking of implementing this system. The questions have been grouped according to whichever of the four elements of Primary Nursing the question addresses. Many people seem to want an outside expert to answer these questions, but each department of nursing and, in some cases, each nursing staff has to participate directly in answering them to assure their relevance to that particular group. The best guidance I can give is to answer each question in terms of the patients' needs first, then nurses' needs, and to do nothing which violates your common sense.

Case Method of Assignment

1. What does case method of assignment mean?
2. How could it work on this unit?
3. What task limits are imposed by job descriptions? Are they necessary and definable limits? For example:
   - Do LPN's pass meds?
   - Regulate IV's?
   - Add IV meds?
   - Who should transcribe and verify physicians' orders?
   - Will Aides carry a patient care assignment?
   - If so, who will supervise and provide back-up?
4. When the case method is used, what kinds of communication support systems are appropriate? Temperature board, Intake and Output summary sheet, assignment work sheet, etc.?

5. What criteria for daily assignments should be used? Rank the criteria identified according to their importance. (List should include, but not be limited to, acuity of patient conditions, skill levels, workload and room location.)

6. How will case method work on the 3-11 and 11-7 shift at the current staffing level? What effect will that have on Primary Nursing?

Twenty-Four-Hour-a-Day Responsibility

1. What does twenty-four-hour-a-day responsibility actually mean?

2. How can that be handled on this station?

3. When the Primary Nurse is off duty, under what types of circumstances should the care plan be changed? What effect, if any, will this have on her authority?

4. Do staff nurses consistently use nursing process? Is any help needed in increasing their comfort level with this activity? Are nursing histories well done when staffing permits? Are the history and care plan forms well designed? Should they be modified for Primary Nursing?

5. Is discharge planning routinely done? How about when census is down and staffing is adequate? What role do staff nurse's perform in discharge planning? Is patient teaching a routine part of daily care? What kinds of support will help the staff perform this activity better?

6. Under what circumstances might it be appropriate to: a) reassign a patient to a new Primary Nurse, and b) to assign daily care to someone other than the Primary Nurse even though she is on duty?

7. Should permanent 3-to-l1 and 11-to-7 nurses ever be Primary Nurses? How can communication with other members of the health team be handled?

8. If the majority of the Primary Nurses work the day shift, how can Primary Nursing be said to exist around the clock?

9. Is the clinical resource information available to the staff appropriate to its needs? If not, what should be added?

10. In addition to the full-time registered nurses, who else can reasonably be expected to function as Primary Nurses? (If part-time nurses are being considered, the question centers on how many consecutive days are worked. If LPN's are being considered, the question centers on their ability and willingness.)

Communication Patterns

1. Is the principle of direct person-to-person communication well accepted by all members of the staff? By the head nurse?

2. Are there individuals uncomfortable with the thought of communicating directly with other nurses at shift report? With doctors? With relatives of patients, or members of other departments? What kinds of assistance would help these individuals?

3. How should shift report be handled?

4. Do guidelines currently exist for presenting information at report? If not, who should develop these guidelines? Should a tape recorder be used? Walking rounds? Face-to-face report? How long should report take? Who should be present?

5. How often should patient care conferences be held? For what purpose? Who should call a conference? Who should conduct it?
6. Who should transcribe physician orders? How should a nurse be notified of new orders?

Role of the Head Nurse

1. How can the head nurse be most helpful to the staff in Primary Nursing?
2. How can she best monitor the quality of care being administered ?
3. Should the head nurse take patients? Should she be a Primary Nurse or work as an Associate to a Primary Nurse when off duty?
4. Should there be a charge nurse with overall responsibility for station-wide decision-making on each shift? Prepare a statement describing the role of the charge nurse.
5. Prepare a statement describing the role of the head nurse and Primary Nurse.

As soon as the staff have answered to their own satisfaction the first three or four questions under case method of assignment, that phase of the implementation process can be undertaken. Task limitations that exist by job description may or may not pose serious constraints on the implementation of case method. Differences in what aides and LPNs are permitted to do vary widely from hospital to hospital. (Some variations are geographical, others exist within the same community, and some, indeed, within the same hospital.) Hospitals where LPNs have traditionally administered medications and where clerical staff have already been transcribing orders will probably find little need to adjust job descriptions as they move from task-based to case-based assignments. Of all the questions listed under case method, the one about job descriptions is the one most likely to require department-wide and perhaps hospital-wide attention. Even though a station staff will not have the final authority to determine task limits set by job descriptions, their recommendations must receive careful attention and thoughtful consideration by those who will be making that decision, and deliberate communication of the staff's solidarity will help assure this.

The group's participation in answering the question about criteria for daily assignment should have an overall beneficial effect on morale. Resentment can be generated by perceived inequities in assignments. Participation in determining the criteria for assignments can provide a non-emotional forum for discussion that can lead to greater understanding and provide the opportunity to resolve old negative feelings. When everyone understands the ground rules and when those rules are applied fairly, ill feelings about workload inequities are eliminated.

Communication pattern changes can be started during the first phase of case assignment. Inadequate communication skills have been one of the largest road blocks to overcome in implementing Primary Nursing. Many individuals experience discomfort in communicating with other members of the health team, particularly with physicians. Others feel unprepared to report off at the end of the shift. Guidelines for shift report may need to be developed to help the inexperienced nurse with this communications requirement. These typically consist of a simple listing of the sequence of patient data to be followed in giving the report. Assertiveness classes have been very helpful in teaching nurses how to communicate effectively with other members of the health team (particularly physicians).

The acquisition of communication skills is an ongoing process. The two types of problems listed above are some that this author has frequently encountered. Feelings of inadequacy and apprehension due to insecurity should be identified early in the process of implementation. Changes in the communication patterns are critical to the successful implementation of Primary Nursing. Appropriate educational resources need to be made available as soon as learning needs are identified.

As the work of answering the above listed questions proceeds concrete changes are occurring simultaneously. Some typical ones are:

1. Elimination of the team leader role assignment, which has the immediate effect of adding two care givers on each day's assignment sheet.
2. Development of new criteria for assigning patients based on skills of the staff members and on the care needs of patients.
3. Expansion of duties may occur, as with LPNs learning to pass medications. Nurses' Aides may realize either expansion or contraction of their patient care responsibility, depending on their particular circumstances. Clerical personnel may likewise experience changes in their roles.
4. Check lists and other systems for handling information are examined for their usefulness when assignments are based on patients rather than tasks. For example: Is a temperature sheet listing all patients' temperatures needed when each nurse takes and records the temperatures of her own patients? (Some hospitals have decided "yes" and others "no.")
5. Identification of clinical learning needs begins. Without exception, taking this step has always resulted in requests from the staff for additional clinical resource material. The need to know more about the sicknesses for which their patients are being treated is always experienced at this time.

The length of time different groups stay at this step varies considerably. The right length of time is however long it takes the staff to become comfortable with the workflow adjustments. This has been as short as two weeks and as long as six months. In a few cases the decision was made to stay at this level of implementation indefinitely. That is O.K. When there are immovable impediments to the further implementation of Primary Nursing, acceptance of case method as the alternative choice may well be the wisest course. As case method implementation proceeds, dialogues, conversations, staff meetings, and conferences about Primary Nursing should be continuing. The more honest sharing of feelings and widespread participation in the decision making process there is at this time, the more interpersonal relationships will be improved. This process often has the effect of tightening the group's bonds and increasing the overall cohesiveness of the staff.

The agreement to implement the major element of the system (the allocation of responsibility) should be made when the staff is ready to do so. The third step of the process is completely taken when each patient has been assigned to a Primary Nurse. Two ways this can be accomplished are to assign all the patients at one time or to do so gradually, over a period of time. I prefer the former approach because I have often observed that a gradual implementation results in a permanently partial implementation.

This decision should be made at a point as near to a complete consensus as possible. If a few individuals are resistant they should be asked to give the system an honest try for a six month period. Most people are willing to try a new idea for at least a limited time. Anyone completely unwilling to agree to try the system even under these circumstances probably ought to be advised to transfer to another situation. Maximum group cohesiveness is highly desirable and will have a strong influence on the outcome of the effort. The earlier emphasis on group participation in the decision making process will have laid the necessary foundation for achieving unity at this time. Cohesiveness among the different groups and shifts provides the atmosphere of support that is vitally important in the risk taking which is a part of Primary Nursing. In fact, this system involves a double risk: that inherent in any decision making situation (if there were no chance of failure it would hardly be a decision making situation) and that of the visible responsibility acceptance demanded by Primary Nursing. In this context, the importance of staff cohesiveness cannot be overemphasized.

Consensus

Staff cohesiveness and decision making by consensus can be achieved in more than one way. The technique that I have used with greatest success is off duty, off premise meetings. Usually these are evening meetings scheduled far enough ahead so necessary arrangements can be made by those who wish to attend. Attendance at these meetings is usually very high, if not at first, certainly by the second or third session. Someone's home is the usual setting; I have probably had some twenty to thirty meetings at my own home and have attended another ten to fifteen in other homes over the years. Often the first meeting is held just prior to the final decision about implementation. The agenda preparation and leadership of the discussion is usually handled by the head nurse. There is no reason, however, why these functions cannot be fulfilled by someone else on the station, or from elsewhere in the organization.

The decision to implement may or may not be a foregone conclusion. If the decision is affirmative, the date for implementation and the steps remaining to be taken will be identified and discussed. How communications about Primary Nursing to appropriate individuals, departments and groups should be handled at this time may also be on the agenda. All of these decisions and discussions may, of course, take place in a wide variety of settings; an off duty, off premise meeting is only one of them, but it has repeatedly proven successful.

Part of the reason for its success is that such meetings are, at one and the same time, part work and part social event, and give the staff a chance to catch up on work-related as well as personal news. It is vitally important for the evening and night staffs to attend these meetings. The identity of all staff members as one group is enhanced in this way. Intershift rivalries and tensions can be dealt with much more effectively in this kind of setting as opposed to change of shift time when tempers can be short. Thus key representatives of all shifts and all categories of workers should be urged to attend these meetings. All station personnel must know that they are or can be members of the group that is deciding how to apply Primary Nursing. Off duty, off premise meetings were used so effectively by some groups I have worked with that they became regular features of station life.

Morale

Inadequate attention to tensions between subgroups, cliques, or factions during this period can effectively impede implementation. Smoldering resentments, long standing jealousies, excessive valuing of credentials over experience, and negative, punitive communication patterns need to be addressed and either eliminated or minimized. Unless the staff is willing to deal with differences of opinion in a supportive, honest, nondestructive manner it will be difficult, if not impossible, to establish the trust between staff members necessary to Primary Nursing. The essence of the system is one nurse with authority over other nurses for the care of her patients. That authority cannot (and probably should not) exist in an atmosphere where people do not trust one another. Unless one nurse has authority over others and her clinical competence is trusted, continuity of nursing care between shifts cannot be maintained. The participative decision making process that has been in use throughout the implementation process will, it is hoped, have had the effect of improving interpersonal relations to the point where disagreements about approaches to patient care can be dealt with maturely and openly.

Visibility

Psychologically, the most difficult part of Primary Nursing occurs now, when the name of the Primary Nurse is put in a place where it will be visible to everyone in the system. Some hospitals use a magnetic board at the desk area to show patient location, physician's name and nurse's name. Others put the name of the nurse on the bed card alongside the names of the physician and the patient. Others put it on the front of the chart, and on the care plan. There is no one right place; the name must simply be put wherever maximum visibility will be achieved.

The success or failure of Primary Nursing often turns on how the staff feels about this phase of implementation, because deep-seated uneasiness about taking risks may surface at this stage, although it will seldom, if ever, be the stated reason for slowing down the implementation. The staff members will probably not consciously recognize this as their basic problem, and will instead cite some of the more typical problems of Primary Nursing. The most popular reason given for the system's not working is inadequate staffing. Others typically include an inadequate drug delivery system, the wrong mixture of personnel, etc. A careful and dispassionate analysis of a breakdown in the system usually reveals a perceived lack of safety on the part of the staff in accepting the risks of having their names published as the individuals responsible for particular patients.

The elements necessary for group members to deal successfully with loss of anonymity and to accept the risks of visible decision making are:

1. Establishment of trust with the members of the work group, especially between day, evening, and night shifts, and between RNs, LPNs and aides.
2. Acceptance of the fact of human error and understanding that mistakes can occur at any level throughout the department of nursing.

Realistic Role Development

The first time a nurse tells a patient she is the Primary Nurse can, for some, be a difficult step. Support, sharing and encouragement among staff nurses can really help in getting over the rough spots. Adequate time and attention must be devoted to dealing with these feelings.

After nurses become comfortable telling patients, physicians and others about being Primary Nurses, certain role developments usually occur. These may have been anticipated by the kinds of inservice education programs usually given to prepare nurses in advance for implementation, but I have found that no amount of formal in-service education is anywhere nearly as effective as the development that takes place spontaneously after the system has been put into practice.

This development normally involves three phases. The first is a desire to know more about the disease processes and medical programs of the patients. Frequently, just after implementation, nurses will begin asking for medical reference textbooks and inservice programs about the physical problems their patients are experiencing. I have frequently found at this stage that medical lectures are most effective and welcome.

The next phase centers on the development of nursing process skills. After nurses become reasonably comfortable in talking about their new roles and feel knowledgeable about the physiological and therapeutic complexities of their patients' conditions, they frequently feel the need to become more proficient care planners. Accordingly, they want to become more efficient data collectors and more effective communicators of the decisions they have made.

At this point staff nurses have consistently and repeatedly requested inservice education on nursing care plans, something quite unique in my years of experience. At this point too our historical problems with nursing care plans, as described earlier, must be dealt with head-on. The accumulated guilt over years of inadequate nursing care plans must be thrown out and a new approach adopted. The care plans were not the problem; the real problem has always been lack of coordination of care. The solution which we tried to make work for years (better nursing care plans) was inadequate because their use did not require acceptance of responsibility, and the plans themselves became the goal of care, not a means to improved coordination.

In Primary Nursing, care plans serve two purposes: 1) to communicate information about a patient's problem and program of care to others who need it and 2) to document the fact that the nursing process has been used as the basis of the patient's care. Unfortunately , before the advent of Primary Nursing, the first purpose was seldom realized in practice. Since care plans had been used during student experiences as the basis for clinical grades, their use as a professional communication tool was completely subordinated to their use as documentation. Now that many institutions are also employing them as evidence of the quality of care administered, their original documentary purpose has again become dominant, reinforced by our desires to attain professional status through the establishment of appropriate and adequate accountability mechanisms. This emphasis, however, has been matched by a continuous erosion of their usefulness as a communication tool.

Using nursing care plans primarily as communication tools between professionals tests their true value. In order to enhance their utility in fulfilling this more meaningful function, their structure, organization and format should be streamlined; as it normally stands now they are often cumbersome, awkward and time-consuming, as well as irrelevant to daily practice. In addition, the language typically used in them is often the legalistic jargon fostered in recent years by an exaggerated preoccupation with "nursing and the law." Since this sort of jargon obscures the transfer of information it is self-defeating. Nursing care plans should be written as originally intended, and ought to employ the everyday language of health professionals. If they are viewed primarily as professional communication tools the staff will respond very positively to their newfound uses and usefulness.

In Primary Nursing the emphasis in care plans is clear. They must contain, first, *the clinical information others need* to care for a patient and, second, *the nursing care instructions written by the Primary Nurse for others to follow* in caring for her patient when she is off duty. These two types of information are essential. It is possible to make sure other nurses know these things through means other than writing them on the care plan (the Primary Nurse can attend report around the clock, phone in each shift, or trust others to convey accurate messages verbally) but most often in Primary Nursing the care plan is the simplest effective communication tool that can be used once the necessary changes in attitude have taken place. As one staff nurse said

> The main problem is when we get low on staff and then the problem isn't with Primary Nursing, it's with trying to get histories and physicals done. We know it ourselves but the care plans aren't done. It's not documented and written so we pass it along at report. And so people really are very conscientious about passing along what they know at the shift time.

When data collection, decision making and written communication of decisions are skills nurses are more comfortable with, nursing care plans improve automatically and dramatically. In Primary Nursing directors no longer have to say, "Joint Commission is coming" in order to assure the writing of care plans because it becomes demonstrably advantageous to the individuals using them to do so.

The third phase of role development in Primary Nursing is the acquisition of communication techniques that enable a nurse to interact more effectively with physicians, relatives of patients and other members of the health team. Again, it is fruitless to try to teach these skills until the other phases of role development have been addressed. Until the Primary Nurse is really convinced that she knows enough (about the patient, the disease, the nursing care, family, relatives or whatever) to deserve the respectful attention of others, she may be unwilling or unable to learn how to articulate her patient's needs to those who need to know. The most troublesome aspect of communication for most nurses is learning "how to talk to God"—the physician. It is not accidental that many nurses feel that this is primarily *what head nurses are paid to do*, but in Primary Nursing this is a "hang up" they will have to get over. Courses in communication, such as assertiveness training programs, can enforce a nurse's self-confidence, thus enabling her to take the risks sometimes inherent in direct communication with some physicians. Group support and encouragement are also important in helping the more reticent nurses develop these skills.

These three phases of development: 1) increased knowledge of medical problems; 2) enhanced nursing process skills and 3) the ability to communicate effectively usually follow one another in a natural progression. Some nurses may need more help with certain developments than others. Nursing administration needs to recognize and accept the fact that the individual nurse is responsible for initiating her own growth and development, but should be ready to provide appropriate educational resources and psychological support as necessary to facilitate that development.

As this third step in the implementation process the agreement to and commencement of the "trial run" gets underway, no great expectations should be laid on the staff. I personally view this as a time of adjustment when the staff have to sort out for themselves what they want to say to patients, relatives and physicians about their new role responsibilities. Care plans, beautiful histories, and elaborate discharge plans can all come later. It is enough at this stage for the nurses to deal with their new visibility and the great challenges and opportunities of their new professional relationships.

Evaluation is the final step in the process. Initially, an informal evaluation is appropriate and adequate. Subjective responses to the change by both staff and patients will be of the greatest value in judging its genuine success.

After the system has been in effect for at least six months, whether or not its original goals have been met should be determined. A simple and effective way to accomplish this is to reissue the questions the staff were asked to answer at the beginning of the implementation process. Usually the planning group is re-formed for this task, and its members collect and summarize the answers (which may be either written or verbal). A report to the whole staff summarizing individual staff members' responses to the four groups of questions can then be made. If the implementation has been wholly successful, this will be a very affirmative experience. The following are some typical reactions:

> I just think it's really neat to have a job that gives you the kind of satisfaction that I've gotten from my relationships with primary patients.

> I'm treated more like a professional person in Primary Nursing, say 80% or 90% of the time, than I ever was in team nursing.

> Here on our floor Primary Nurses are promoting patient care and themselves as professional people and everybody is beginning to recognize that. Primary Nurses really care about patients and are more professional.

> I think Primary Nursing has actually caused the team of the doctor and the nurse to work better together. We're a lot closer today and I think the doctors really do respect us a lot more. I can't believe how many times the doctor now discusses things with me.

The hard core of the evaluation must be the staff's perception of its success or failure. If difficulties still exist with the implementation of Primary Nursing, this evaluation process will serve to focus attention on the problem so that it can be defined and solutions sought by appropriate staff members.

At the very minimum, the evaluation requires the participation of all members of the nursing staff. A much wider assessment is often made in which the reactions of patients, physicians and other members of the health team are sought. These can be acquired in interviews, by questionnaire or by the solicitation of testimonials. In many hospitals the approach is much more formal, but regardless of its design the subjective opinions of the staff must be solicited and the effect they perceive the system to have had on their patients must be determined. It is the obligation of each and every person entrusted to care for the sick to make sure that that care is being rendered in the best way possible. Thus, whatever else it may include and whoever participates in it, the evaluation of the system must ultimately be made in terms of its impact on patients.

Addendum to Chapter Four

After years of teaching this transformational process, I am convinced it is one of the most powerful ways to change culture and empower staff. As I have continued my experiential study, I realize it is a group dynamic process using the energy of both positive and negative informal leaders within the staff. The marvelous outcome is that the implementation process provides the "culture media" for developing staff's decision-making skills as well as teaching them effective ways to improve interpersonal relationships. Every group has positive and negative leaders; that is, people who encourage others in positive or negative attitudes about changes, work, administration and the unit. Primary Nursing brings these informal leaders together with a specific set of decisions they are empowered to make, and requires them to become an effective, healthy group. These core influencers have an opportunity to experience the coming operational change and learn how to deal with it in advance.

Since Primary Nursing gives each staff nurse the right and responsibility to make decisions about the nursing care of a small group of patients, the core leaders have an opportunity to experience making decisions about the way the unit operates. A large part of decision-making is experiencing the consequences of those decisions, whether clinical or operational. This process sets the stage for staff to experience that at the level of unit operations.

In order for one nurse to be responsible for decision-making about the care of a patient, interpersonal relationships have to be better than in any other system. Teamwork has to be much better in Primary Nursing than it ever had to be in team nursing. This method of implementation gives the informal leaders an opportunity to experience decision-making and managing healthy relationships in preparation for the system change. Because they are the leaders, bringing the rest of the staff on board is much easier than if they have had no influence.

The process used in the fourth chapter can be used to empower any work group, if it is followed with attention to the important elements.

The Delegation of Authority

When the idea of decision-making at the level of action is embraced, careful thought needs to be given to the level at which it is appropriate to delegate. It is the responsibility of top leadership to define the nature of the change and the parameters of the decisions to be made at each level. I have always believed the decision to go to Primary Nursing is one that legitimately belongs to the chief nurse, where rests the responsibility and authority to set the standards of practice for the department.

Because the system is based on the philosophy of decentralized decision-making, the trick lies in appropriately designing the process of implementation. Primary Nursing fails miserably whenever the chief nurses say, "Ve vill do Primary Nursing because I say so, and I am zee Boss!" Au contraire! I have seen some spectacular implementations fail when the change is approached in this manner. Rather, the chief nurse needs to set the standard—i.e.: each patient's care will be managed by a single RN throughout his or her stay on a unit—and design an implementation program consistent with the principle of decentralized decision-making.

Leadership Development

The administrative and managerial support structure must be changed to facilitate the development of professional practice at the unit level. Managers control and leaders develop. In a professional practice setting, leadership rather than management is the requirement.

During the seventies while I was functioning as chief nurse at United Hospitals in St. Paul, Minnesota and Yale New Haven in Connecticut, I came to understand how important the role of the nurse manager was to the success of Primary Nursing. In fact, once in each hospital I actually approved the "un-implementation" of Primary Nursing when I realized the manager was incapable of giving up control over patient care. It became even more clear to me during the seventies as hospitals all over the country began to bill themselves as doing Primary Nursing—usually in recruitment ads. As I came to learn, a typical pattern was that it would be established on one or two units, then the implementation stopped. Upon inquiring why it hadn't been implemented further, the common answer was that these were the one or two best units with the greatest morale and strongest leaders in the nurse manager role. As I put the experience with my own two nurse managers into context, I came to realize that in order for this system to work, the typical role of the nurse managers had to change. This is a necessity, not just a nice change.

In 1982 I developed the first coordinated curriculum for nurse managers based on sound theories and constructed in a way that transformed their understanding of their role, as well as provided them the tools they needed to become leaders. Originally constructed as a five-day program, including a day and a half on staffing, it was later reduced to three days and is now delivered and licensed throughout the United States and internationally. This program—now called LEO for Leading an Empowered Organization—is primarily offered to front-line managers within an institution. Its relevance is widely recognized for all disciplines and departments.

Implementation Process Decisions

The real breakthrough in successfully replicating Primary Nursing came as I learned a practical and effective way to give the staff the right and responsibility to make decisions about how the system will operate on their unit. This required careful delineation of the principals of clinical decision-making authority, work allocation, communication and management. They were clearly defined. The definition of those organization elements has to be differentiated clearly among the four prototypical delivery systems—functional, team, total, and Primary Nursing. Only then can decision-making be safely delegated to staff to decide how those elements will operate on their own unit. Over the years we learned this is best accomplished with a set of carefully worded questions that require discussion, dialog and finally, decisions. The wording may vary depending on the current reality, but the model questions used in the fourth chapter should guide their construction. The answers to the questions must become implementation decisions! Otherwise the discussion may be purely academic. Take as an example the question "When is it appropriate to change a Primary Nurse's care plan when she is off duty?" and the corollary: "What effect will this have on the Primary Nurse's authority?" As staff members think through various scenarios in response to these questions, they are developing implementation guidelines. The process requires a consensus-based outcome and therefore the quality of the answer is usually excellent.

To support the implementation of a professional practice care delivery model, Creative Health Care Management developed an implementation guide for use with clients. The introduction to that implementation guide creates a cohesive and comprehensive frame of reference for considering all the issues involved in creating a professional practice care delivery system. The introduction to this guide is included as an appendix to this book (see appendix B).

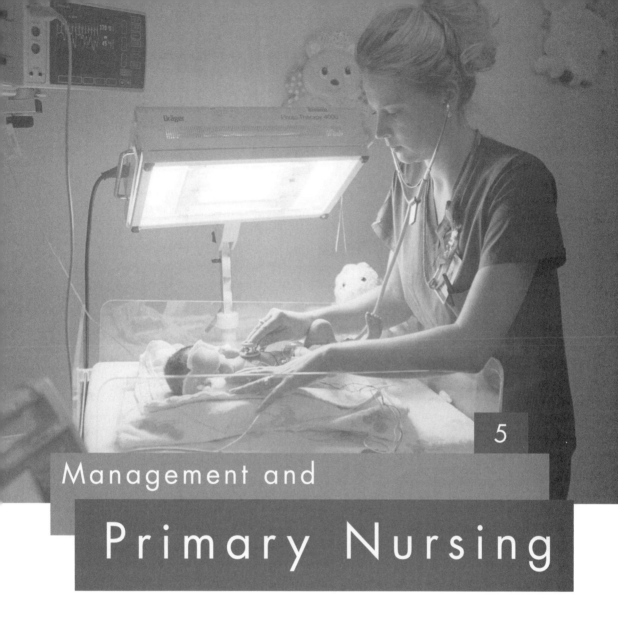

5

Management and
Primary Nursing

The implementation process described in the preceding chapter was a more or less isolated phenomenon. It can occur once within a given hospital, or it can occur repeatedly; it can remain a localized experiment or become the foundation of an entire hospital's care system. There are many factors that determine how widespread the implementation of Primary Nursing will be in any given institution. The three most important are: 1) the organizational theory on which the existing administrative structure is founded; 2) the attitude of management toward Primary Nursing; and 3) the functions of management in the implementation process.

Organizational Theory and Administrative Structure

The organizational theory that provides the best foundation for Primary Nursing is decentralized decision making. As illustrated in previous chapters, it means simply the granting of decision making authority to those at the level of action, who are in the best position to judge the adequacy and efficacy of the decisions they make. Decentralization of this authority has the effect of flattening hierarchies. It recognizes the value of individuals within all levels, putting them in control of their own actions and (to a somewhat lesser extent) the environment in which those actions take place. Each individual is answerable for the consequences of his actions; accountability is the flip side of the responsibility coin.

In *People or Personnel* by Paul Goodman [15] the difference between centralized and decentralized decision making management philosophies is explained and the types of institutions or organizations that ought to be organized around the different management theories are categorized. He recommends centralized management decision making in institutions or organizations where the product of the functions performed is inanimate and where the tasks used to accomplish the functions are repetitive, mechanistic, automatic, and predictable. In institutions or organizations where the product is a human being, however, and the tasks used to accomplish the functions are neither repetitious, automatic nor predictable, he recommends the use of decentralized decision making. The human being in the hospital is never perfectly predictable and Goodman goes on to say specifically that such institutions ought to be organized around the theory of decentralized decision making.

There are three elements in the theory that need to be taken apart, examined separately as they affect each level of authority in the hierarchy of a department of nursing, and then reassembled into a cohesive administrative structure. These three elements are:

1. The clear allocation and acceptance of responsibility for decision making.
2. The delegation to an individual of authority which is commensurate with her responsibility.
3. The establishment of mechanisms of accountability so that the quality of the decisions that have been made can be evaluated.

The absence of these three elements in the hierarchy of the department of nursing will deter the implementation of Primary Nursing.

In Primary Nursing decentralization means bringing decision making to the bedside. A nurse needs and is given responsibility for the nursing care received by a patient around the clock, seven days a week. She is authorized to direct the actions of other nurses who care for her patients when she is not there, which presupposes their respect and trust of her as essential ingredients in their interpersonal relationships. Mechanisms of accountability therefore need to be established so that the quality of her decisions as Primary Nurse can be examined to determine whether or not good clinical judgment is being used. Currently, the head nurse in most hospitals provides whatever accountability there is in the system. However, quality assurance programs are being developed in some hospitals that enable a staff nurse's decision making process to be measured against standards of practice that have been established by other staff nurses. The development of these programs based on standards of practice set by peers elevates our practice to a higher level of professionalism than it previously had. Peer review without being able to identify single decision makers is impossible and therefore necessitates decentralization of decision making to the staff nurse level. It can thus be the first step in the development of a professional practice of nursing within the bureaucratic setting of the hospital.

The importance of a consistent approach to decision making throughout the administrative structure of the department cannot be overemphasized. In Primary Nursing, staff nurses are being asked to take the risk of visibility in their decision making. If the same degree of visible responsibility acceptance does not exist in the higher levels of the hierarchy, the staff nurses are likely to feel vulnerable on the one hand, and to lack trust and confidence in their superiors on the other. If individuals in superior positions will not accept, with visibility, the risks of making mistakes in management decisions, how can the staff nurse be expected to accept the risks of mistake making in clinical practice? It is very important that the responsibilities of all levels of the hierarchy be clarified and that authority be delegated accordingly. A good test of whether or not there is clear understanding of levels of responsibility and authority is to ask individuals to describe their own jobs in these terms, as well as the jobs of their immediate superiors and subordinates. If people are holding positions that they cannot describe in a way that others can understand, then a major position definition and clarification effort is called for.

A centralized decision making structure should be decentralized in order to support the implementation of Primary Nursing. It is difficult (not impossible, but very difficult) for it to be successfully implemented when management decision making remains highly centralized. A reasonable timetable (not longer than six months) should be targeted for this reorganization process.

An administrative structure that supports Primary Nursing must be assessed according to two criteria. The first is the degree of congruity between responsibility, authority and accountability at all levels of authority within the superstructure and the second is whether or not twenty-four-hour-a-day responsibility for patient care exists at appropriate levels within the organization.

There are only three or four natural levels of authority within any department of nursing from bedside nurse to director of nursing. The first is the Primary Nurse who has responsibility and authority for the care of a group of patients and the second is the head nurse who has responsibility and authority over the quality of care administered to an entire group of patients. In large hospitals there is usually a third level, a position of many titles. Here, for the sake of simplicity, I will just call it the "middle management level." The fourth level of authority within the department is, of course, that of the director of nursing who is responsible and has the authority and is held accountable for the quality of care administered throughout the institution by all members of the nursing department at all times.

To determine whether or not responsibility, authority and accountability are properly matched at the various levels of the department of nursing, a few key questions can be asked. For example: 1) Will other nurses follow the care plan of the Primary Nurse? If the Primary Nurse does not have authority over the nurses who care for her patients in her absence, then she cannot be held responsible for the quality of care a patient receives on a twenty-four-hour-a-day basis. 2) Does the head nurse take the blame from a physician when a lab report is not on the chart, thus implying that she can be held responsible for something over which she has no authority? Not until the head nurse designs the lab reporting system will it be appropriate for her to accept the blame for its failure. 3) Can the supervisor of a particular area select a head nurse on her service? 4) Does the director of nursing need to ask permission from the hospital administrator or chief of the medical staff in order to implement Primary Nursing? If she does not have the authority to develop improvements in the delivery system used for nursing care she cannot legitimately be held responsible for its quality. Honest answers to these questions will help indicate the degree of congruence between responsibility and authority.

The second criterion is the clear allocation of twenty-four-hour-a-day responsibility at the head nurse and middle management levels of a department to ensure that adequate continuity between the shifts is successfully maintained. This is an area where lip service and reality are often inconsistent. If the head nurse does not have primary responsibility for the evaluation of the permanent 3 to 11 and 11 to 7 floor personnel, then she does not have twenty-four-hour-a-day responsibility for the floor. The importance of this criterion cannot be overemphasized.

A special word is in order about the middle manager, the congruence of whose authority and responsibility is often the most out of line. Most commonly called the supervisors, they have a range of titles that runs the gamut from director to coordinator. Over the past ten years, this role has perhaps changed the most (or at least been threatened the most) and is still the least clearly defined. The dichotomy between administration and clinical practice is felt most exquisitely by individuals in this position. They are continually given more responsibility for administration, and yet many institutions seem to expect them to maintain a high degree of clinical expertise as well. So often they are the individuals called by other nurses when a special clinical problem requires expert handling but in fact they are often the last to know of advances in medical technology because they are so preoccupied with administrative problems. (It is only in the past ten years that people have stopped expecting the director of nursing to step into complex clinical situations as the in-house expert. Most directors no longer even wear uniforms.) Changes in others' expectations of middle managers have, unfortunately, gone in one direction only: an increase in administrative involvement with no lessening in expectations of their clinical skills. This has often left these middle managers the most frustrated and insecure in the nursing family. Nevertheless, their attitude toward Primary Nursing is of importance second only to that of the head nurse, whose successful leadership in implementing Primary Nursing will often depend on the middle manager's support and a tolerant attitude toward the risk taking of decision making.

The Attitude of the Members of the Management Team

The second vital factor affecting implementation of Primary Nursing is the attitude of the management team. If its members start out with a firm belief that most nurses want to take good care of their patients, and if they adopt an attitude of support without pressure, the implementation process will be greatly facilitated and its chances for complete success vastly enhanced.

The adoption by the management team of a philosophy of support without force is of fundamental importance to the system. Primary Nursing cannot be implemented by management edict; it must be implemented by the staff of a station. This is often difficult for individuals in positions of authority to accept. For me personally it was extraordinarily difficult since my belief in Primary Nursing knows no boundaries. Since 1969, my life has been dedicated to the implementation of this system but I have had to accept, albeit reluctantly, the fact that I cannot just *make* nurses into Primary Nurses. That acceptance has been reinforced by the recognition that there are certain types of people who, if they are pressured into this system against their will, can subtly (and sometimes not-so-subtly) sabotage it in ways that will endanger not only its success but patient safety as well. The only way I know to avoid this kind of aggravating and destructive behavior is to insist on these individuals' participation in the decision making process. This will help make their actions public and their responsibility for them visible, and it will also help the individuals become more conscious of their own motivations. The important thing is that they come to see their participation as voluntary, even if it is only on a trial basis.

In my Preface I expressed my strong belief that virtually all nurses are motivated by a sincere desire to give good nursing care. This belief is essential among managers because of two important attitudes to which it gives rise. The first is that since nurses *want* to give good nursing care, few controls are necessary to prevent willful wrong doing. Excessive use of management control mechanisms communicates to the staff an expectation that if not controlled they will perform in undesirable ways. This negative approach by management results in people feeling as if they are being treated like little children, which encourages them to act that way.

The second is an attitude of tolerance toward human error. The fear of committing errors in the treatment of patients has led us into thinking of mistake making as aberrant or unnatural. Although a supreme being is presumed to be the only entity to whom we may attribute infallibility, the profession of nursing has not learned how to deal effectively with the simple, basic reality of human fallibility. From its beginning nursing has dealt with human frailty by punishment. (One wonders why society keeps trying to use punishment to control behavior when such great evidence of its ineffectiveness surrounds us daily.) When nursing was task-oriented the nature of a mistake was quite different than it is now that we are judgment-oriented. The nature of making a procedural mistake is quite unlike making a mistake in clinical judgment. The traditional swift and severe punishment for the former has impeded our ability to accept the mistake making inherent in the exercise of clinical judgment.

Why is mistake making inherent in this kind of judgment? Clinical nursing judgment is used to solve problems the patient presents based on the knowledge and the experience the nurse brings to the assessment of the situation. The basic steps of the decision making process are used by the nurse and the activity is called "the nursing process." What we have failed to deal with in teaching nursing process is the reality that a nurse will usually have to make a decision about a problem *before* she has had time to acquire all of the relevant information. This means that at least some of the time a wrong decision will be made because the information on which it was based was *inadequate*. We foster the myth that decision making is based on adequate data collection, but in the real world there is seldom time to do the literature search, thorough family interview, complete physical assessment, etc., required for completely adequate data collection. Clinical decision making must consequently admit to the possibility of error. But our knee-jerk reaction to any mistake has been punishment; our earliest reaction was to expel the wrongdoer. By the late forties and fifties a student nurse who had committed an error was forced to appear in the hospital without her cap. Today, evaluations, audit reports, conferences and incident reports are sometimes used as a more subtle form of punishment.

A management team must deal with the emotional backwash of this punishment-oriented heritage. As already described, one of the most serious impediments to the successful implementation of Primary Nursing is the pure fear staff nurses feel when confronted with the requirement that their names appear on the front of their patients' charts. The initial response is frequently "My God, he'll know who to yell at." Members of the management team must deal openly with this problem and discuss their attitudes toward mistake making. A good exercise to start with is for each member of the management team to discuss a serious error in practice she committed in her first staff nurse position. This telegraphs the important message to the bedside nurse that management acknowledges, understands and accepts the risk taking element of decision making. If the superiors have taken risks and admitted to human errors the Primary Nurse will feel safer and the atmosphere in which the system is being tried out will be healthier.

The two factors affecting the ease with which Primary Nursing can be implemented—the theories of organization most conducive to its success and the most desirable attitudes on the part of management—are certainly important to the final outcome, but it should be noted that they are not essential. I have seen the system implemented in settings where the atmosphere, especially at the upper levels, was not at all hospitable. Primary Nursing can be implemented in spite of this; it simply requires more courageous staff nurses.

Functions of Management in Implementing Primary Nursing

Once agreement has been reached to try out Primary Nursing whether or not the decision has been unanimous, or made by a group of staff nurses, or by individuals higher up in the nursing administration hierarchy; and whether or not the theoretical basis of the organization and the attitude of management toward the experiment are favorable individuals at the management level must take certain steps if they wish the system to have a fair trial. The following are the most effective facilitative mechanisms I have seen used in various hospitals:

1. Internal assessment of the effectiveness of the administrative structure.
2. Appointment of a central committee for Primary Nursing.
3. Appointment of an individual to coordinate implementation.
4. The establishment of a Primary Nursing Advisory Council.

Putting these mechanisms into effect calls for the contributions of various managers.

The Role of the Director of Nursing

The internal assessment of administrative efficacy has been discussed previously, in the last chapter and in the context of organizational theories. It is an area in which the director of nursing can most effectively exert her leadership by seeing to it that necessary preconditions are met:

1. Administrative support of the concept of continuous operational responsibility, clearly allocated so everyone knows who is responsible for what and when.
2. The matching of responsibility with a commensurate degree of authority for individuals at all levels of the department.

3. A philosophy of tolerance in regard to (reasonable) errors in clinical judgment, sufficient to permit necessary risk taking.

The director of nursing must not only see that these conditions exist but must also be able to articulate them to the entire department as an official philosophy, in the fulfillment of which individuals can expect administrative support.

The Central Committee for Primary Nursing

The appointment of a central committee to facilitate implementation on a department-wide basis has been beneficial. Members should include people in key management positions (day, evening, and night may be appropriate), some staff nurses, as well as members of the inservice education department. The chairperson of this committee should be selected for her knowledge and understanding of the entire department of nursing, the hospital as a whole, and the pockets of power that exist within the hospital community. It is important that this chairperson be seen as an agent of the director of nursing (assuming, of course, that the director of nursing supports the implementation of Primary Nursing).

The functions of this committee should include the following:

1. Identification of administrative changes necessary to support Primary Nursing.
2. Recommendation of departmental changes below the administrative level necessary to support the system of Primary Nursing.
3. Identification and dissemination of literature and information about other resources which will help staff at all levels understand and contribute to the implementation of the system.

Examples of activities this committee might perform are:

- A review of the statement of departmental philosophy and objectives to evaluate its appropriateness to Primary Nursing.
- A review of all other departmental and hospital policies affecting the nursing department to determine their appropriateness to Primary Nursing. Inconsistencies (e.g., use of the title "team leader") should be ironed out through liaison with other departments.
- A review of all nursing procedures to determine their appropriateness under the new system.
- A review of job descriptions and their rewriting to make them consistent with the requirements of Primary Nursing.

The Primary Nursing Central Committee may appropriately be empowered to revise, rewrite or establish the statements of policy, procedure, job descriptions, etc. In many hospitals, though, standing committees already exist for these purposes, in which case it is better for them to carry them out. In practice the central committee's main function will be to assess the compatibility of the existing administrative systems with the principles of Primary Nursing.

The Primary Nursing System Coordinator

Some hospitals (including two in which the author was Director of Nursing) have found it useful to designate someone as "Primary Nursing Coordinator" or "Primary Nursing Liaison" (or something similarly descriptive). Usually, one RN can handle this function as an additional assignment over and above her regular tasks and responsibilities (although it may be necessary on a short term basis to reallocate some of her job responsibilities to make time for the new task). While not absolutely necessary it makes a great deal of sense for this coordinator to be chairperson of the Primary Nursing Central Committee as well. That way, there is one clearly visible person within the organization who serves as a resource to individuals at any level interested in pursuing the concept of Primary Nursing. The individual selected must always be someone in a position of authority that reflects a high value in the organization. It may be a nurse from the inservice education department or someone with special project or research and development responsibilities, or else the nurse with primary responsibility for coordinating discharge referrals. The other responsibilities that this individual holds are not of particular importance. What is of primary importance is that she be well respected by all levels of the nursing staff and be seen as one who understands head nurses and, especially, the station staff.

Both the Primary Nursing Coordinator and a majority of the members of the Central Committee are likely to be drawn from middle management levels. It is entirely appropriate for the director of nursing to expect individuals at this level to deal personally with the issues raised by Primary Nursing. Lack of support at this level can be a sufficient deterrent to prevent its implementation in the areas over which one such individual has influence. If Primary Nursing becomes an accepted goal of the department of nursing then it is reasonable and proper for the director of nursing service to expect support for the concept from the individuals in middle management positions. Sabotage of a department goal is not to be tolerated.

Primary Nursing Advisory Council

Another positive mechanism to facilitate the implementation of Primary Nursing is the establishment of a Primary Nursing Advisory Council. Historically, this council has developed as a loosely organized staff nurse/head nurse meeting where individuals already doing Primary Nursing and those considering it can discuss, *in the absence of their superiors*, the problems and solutions, successes and failures they are experiencing or anticipate experiencing in the new system. (If there is a Primary Nursing Coordinator she too would normally attend sessions of this council, but not in a managerial capacity.) With its primary emphasis on the mutual sharing of experiences the greatest benefit of this council is self-growth through self-help. Since it is not a formal committee of the hospital or department *per se*, its meetings can be kept as informal as participants like. They seem to work best when nursing administration provides a time, place, and advance notification but it should not attempt to direct the meeting, select the people who attend, or hand down solutions to the problems expressed. Ideally, these solutions will come as a natural byproduct of the sharing process. Solutions that require administrative actions can be brought to the attention of nursing administration by the Advisory Council in the form of recommendations, which must receive careful and serious consideration and prompt action from whoever is designated to act on them: the Primary Nursing Central Committee, the Primary Nursing Coordinator, or in many instances, the director of nursing.

To summarize, there are four positive steps that can be taken by a central nursing administration to support and facilitate the successful implementation of Primary Nursing. These are 1) an internal review of administrative structure; 2) the establishment of a Primary Nursing Central Committee charged with seeing that necessary department-wide changes are made to enhance departmental support for the concept of Primary Nursing; 3) the establishment of a Primary Nursing Coordinator or Implementor to help keep the implementation process moving; and 4) the establishment of the Primary Nursing Advisory Council to serve as a forum in which staff nurses and head nurses can share their experiences with the new system.

Popular Myths about Implementation

A few words are in order about approaches to implementation which, after being tried, have been found inadequate. One of these, which this author and others have used with little long-term success, is the establishment of a pilot station. The thinking behind experimenting on a smaller scale seems valid on the surface, but repeated experience with this approach has led me to discourage its use in any hospital that is seriously considering widespread implementation of the system.

When people are facing a change as pervasive as that from team to Primary Nursing, it seems desirable to localize the potential negative effects as much as possible. The risk of failure is not as frightening when it is restricted to a carefully controlled setting. It is assumed that under these circumstances any mistakes made in the implementation process can be more easily corrected, and that others can learn from these mistakes and avoid repeating them. However, these assumptions are founded on the flawed belief that Primary Nursing will thrive when it is imposed and controlled from above. As I have emphasized repeatedly the system is likely to succeed only when a group of nurses who work together plan the implementation. If the staff of two, three, four or more units wish to plan concurrently, there is no reason why they should not do so. Since every staff has the right to decide the question for itself, an attempt to implement the system hospital-wide can be too unwieldy and as unlikely to succeed as a specially designated pilot station. Overall coordination of a multiple-station implementation is not an excessively difficult task. What matters most is that the first station or stations to implement Primary Nursing should select themselves.

The timing of implementation cannot be controlled by the director of nursing or any other individual. Primary Nursing should occur when people feel themselves ready to make the necessary changes required for the system to be put in place. I have visited hospitals where implementation institution-wide is awaiting the collection of before-and-after data from a pilot station while the staffs of other stations have been eminently ready to implement the system and have felt extremely frustrated with the enforced wait. Meanwhile, nurses on the pilot station feel as if they are living in a goldfish bowl, becoming increasingly fatigued and anxious. All in all, the establishment of a pilot station is an "unnatural" approach to implementation, the possible advantages of which are outweighed by the likely disadvantages.

Another popular but ultimately counterproductive approach to implementing Primary Nursing is the prior establishment of a set of *selection criteria* according to which participants in the experimental program will be picked. The underlying assumption seems to be that Primary Nurses have special characteristics, qualifications, educational preparation, or personality attributes that make them different from the average staff nurse. The inescapable destructive effect this has on morale in the nursing department cannot be overemphasized. A corollary of this assumption is that some of the individuals currently employed on the implementation station will be found unqualified to administer nursing in the new system. While criteria are being established and the selection process is getting underway the effect on personal relationships and morale in general is profoundly negative. Nothing is more likely to undermine the cohesiveness of a closely knit work group than being threatened from outside by the elimination of some of its members and the addition of new ones.

I am not suggesting that everyone employed in a particular situation will necessarily be able to perform satisfactorily in Primary Nursing. I stress again, though, that an effectively functioning group which has made a conscious decision to implement Primary Nursing be recognized as the single appropriate milieu for the experiment. If any individual within the group is unable (or, more usually, unwilling) to make a successful adjustment to the new delivery system, the situation can be corrected after Primary Nursing is underway. It has been my experience that with the proper educational opportunities, and strong professional leadership, any individual in a care giving role finds the Primary Nursing system the most comfortable and rewarding way to carry out her job responsibilities.

Finally, there is the myth that Primary Nursing can be taught to nurses before the system is implemented so that on Day One of an implementation everyone has been "adequately prepared" to function in the *role* of Primary Nurse. This misjudgment has caused enormous amounts of frustration and a deep sense of futility in those trying to design a foolproof implementation plan not to mention those who are supposed to carry it out. The truth is that until the system changes the role cannot develop. People cannot learn how to perform on a more professional level of nursing in a setting that rewards only bureaucratic competence. If they could, they would have done so a long time ago. The unique role of the Primary Nurse must develop naturally and, during this process the appropriate function of leadership is to provide educational resources and other support as needed. It is not to assess, identify, define and evaluate those needs, but simply to provide adequate resources. The role will then develop naturally and the truly professional nursing practice dreamed about by millions of nurses over the years will become the everyday reality of patient care.

Addendum to Chapter Five

Twenty years of watching Primary Nursing ebb and flow in institutions through-out the United States and around the world have led me to the conclusion that the challenges of professional, relationship-based, accountable nursing practice require enlightened and skilled leadership at managerial and, we hope, executive levels. Nursing is a very special activity. Vulnerable people. Complex technology. Continuity of care 24/7/365. External regulations. Shortened lengths of stay. Twelve-hours shifts. Combined, these elements create parameters that often seem like barriers to humane, sensitive, caring practice.

Hospital administrators seem to seesaw between decentralization and centralization. Changes in leadership inevitably impact the emphasis on one end or the other of the seesaw. And so it goes with Primary Nursing. When the seesaw tilts toward decentralization and empowerment, professional practice ascends in value, and when administrative philosophy moves toward centralization of power, task-based nursing wins out. Seldom is this discussed as clearly as I am writing about it now. Often rhetoric obfuscates the truth. For example, when skill-mix changes are mandated from above, without regard for the patients' acuity or staff nurses' delegation competence, controls used to implement the new skill mix often drive bedside nurses into a frenzy of task-based practice. In contrast, when skill-mix changes are implemented in a transformational process, professional practice is strengthened.

New leadership, staffing shortages, skill-mix changes, RN cutbacks and a multitude of other realities often negatively affect Primary Nursing. When nursing becomes even more mechanical and task-based, and stressful, staff often remember Primary Nursing with fondness. Then at some point, a decision is made to revise the care-delivery system, and the discussion centers on the good old days. Nurse leaders start rethinking the elements of Primary Nursing, looking for what can be incorporated into their current reality to reignite the awesome spirit of practice so often experienced in a Primary Nursing system.

The Power of R-A-A

What seemed simply like a logical approach to organizing a department along lines consistent with the care-delivery system has turned out to be of enormous value, leading to wonderful clarity of role definitions and a great deal of personal growth. I am referring to the definition of the three elements of decentralization defined on page 58:

1. The clear allocation and acceptance of responsibility for decision making.
2. The delegation to an individual of authority which is commensurate with her responsibility.
3. The establishment of mechanisms of accountability so that the quality of the decisions that have been made can be evaluated.

The language used in those definitions is still highly appropriate. Sociologists say autonomy is an absolute requirement in order for an enterprise to deserve the title of a profession. It is not the only requirement and others are equally important, although not universally agreed to by sociologists—altruism, identifiable body of knowledge, etc. However, for nursing, the other elements have been easier to achieve. It is only now, with Primary Nursing a viable option

67

for hospital nursing practice, that autonomy is recognized as the essential ingredient for hospital nursing to be professional.

In the thirty years since the original implementation, the problem of the nurse's personal power at the bedside has become crystal clear. While discussions of this problem usually center on the complex issues of a dysfunctional health care system—physician power and bureaucratic claptrap—among others, I have become convinced that *the main cause of nurse powerlessness is self-induced*. We are a profession that figuratively stands in place with hands out waiting to be given something that we already own. And that is the authority to prescribe the amount, degree and kind of nursing care a hospitalized patient will receive. The fact that physicians can order medically related activities continues to blur nursing's vision about its own role.

The sheer joy of Primary Nursing is seeing a nurse's vision clear up when she accepts responsibility for managing the care of a specific group of patients and establishes a responsibility-relationship that is clear to the patients, their families, the physicians and the nursing staff. We have all the authority over nursing care we need, yet we seldom experience that authority because we don't engage in the key activity of accepting responsibility visibly and clearly within the system. Authority must be experienced to be known. It is not an intellectual activity that can be taught in a classroom. If it were, we would not have the annual rite of passage that occurs on July 1 in every medical center in the United States: new residents begin to write orders. A similar rite of passage within nursing is the establishment of the responsibility relationship with patients that is visible throughout the system. It is not enough for a nurse to feel responsible for managing a patient's nursing care. Unless the patient and family, nursing staff and other health care disciplines understand the nature of the responsibility relationship the nurse has established with the patient, it doesn't exist. It must be visible in order to be real.

Managing the Transformation

Two other issues need to be addressed in the development of a professional nursing department. Both center on endemic nurse powerlessness. First, leaders need to be empowered and manifest that empowerment to their staffs. When individuals in hierarchical positions feel and act like victims, they reinforce that behavior among the staff. This is especially important at first-level leadership positions. If individuals in these positions behave as if they have no choices, are being whipsawed between administration and staff and victimized into ridiculously long work weeks, the message to the staff is loud and clear. *Victim thinking is part of this culture.* So, a key developmental issue is facilitating an empowered leadership group. This is no easy task, when the worldwide changes keep requiring new responses. Leaders must have strong discernment regarding their own personal responsibilities to maintain a healthy sense of professional autonomy.

The second essential issue is the culture of the unit. This is the almost osmotic communication of norms and mores between staff members. Subcultures even exist between shifts and among categories within a skill mix. Nurse managers, charge nurses and supervisory staff need to be aware of the almost subliminal messages conveyed to the staff about norms and mores and work to change those that are negative or dysfunctional and to reinforce those that are positive and motivating.

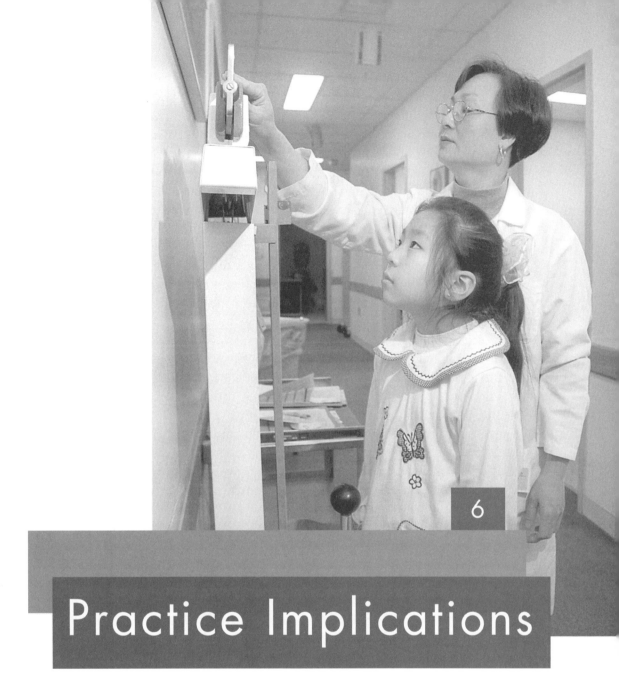

6

Practice Implications

Educational Implications

There are two major educational implications of Primary Nursing, the use of Primary Nurses as teachers, and the place of Primary Nursing in the curriculum.

The clinician/teacher method of nursing education is still considered by many (including the author) to be a superior teaching process. When nursing education and service were separated, use of this model disappeared, and the problems created by the loss have been serious and to a large extent unsolvable. Joint appointments hold some promise of reintegrating education and service by faculty who are both clinicians and teachers, but insofar as such appointments currently exist their usefulness is very limited, particularly at the level of basic education; and are not sufficient to make the clinician/teacher model universal in undergraduate programs.

The proposal I am outlining here recognizes the value of increasing joint appointments and suggests that Primary Nurses, employed by a hospital, be used in a productive way as clinician/teachers for basic nursing education. Consistently positive results have supported my belief that patient presentation by Primary Nurses can, in a relatively short period of time, greatly enhance a student nurse's knowledge of complicated interrelated factors of patient care. A ten to fifteen minute presentation of a diabetic patient that focuses on the interrelated aspects of care in that complicated disease process is a far more effective use of a student nurse's time than is an hour spent giving a diabetic patient a bed bath. It is unrealistic to expect classroom-based faculty to be able to teach a comparable level of clinical judgment. The Primary Nurse is the most logical one to prepare the students for the real complexities of professional nursing practice. Creative and innovative ways to tap this knowledge and make it available to student nurses should be explored by those who are responsible for the education of future nurses.

The curricular implications of Primary Nursing are profound. Teaching decision making is no mean task. The majority of Primary Nurses practicing today must learn this skill on the job. Other professionals acquire it as part of their education; it is appropriate for nurses to do so also.

Decision making cannot be taught in a laboratory. If it could, teaching hospitals would never have been needed for medical education. In order to teach it effectively there must be three risk takers: a faculty member, a student and a patient (whose share of the risk is, ideally, minimal). This is true for both medicine and nursing, the only difference being that medicine has always recognized the essential priority of professional decision making.

Nursing education has not placed a high value on independent decision making by practitioners. Student nurses do not "carry a case load" with any degree of independence even in the final stages of their preparation. Many schools still teach students how to perform as team leaders, but that role actually requires little or no understanding of problem solving or decision making. For example, as team leaders many students are still taught to collect "all the necessary data" before making a decision about a patient's care needs. To do this at all thoroughly requires unrealistic amounts of time and consequently one finds care decisions not being explicitly made because not enough data was collected. In the real world, besides basic clinical decision making skills, students need to learn the realities of priority setting and judicious corner cutting or they will never be able to make important decisions on an hour-by-hour basis during times of busy workloads—a failure which distresses both student and patient.

There are two areas of decision making required of a care giving nurse. The first is deciding how to care for a particular patient and the second is coordinating such care for a number of patients. Clinical decision making ability and management decision making ability are both called for. Managing a case load of patients requires planning, including priority setting, performing the care and evaluating its effectiveness. In order to accomplish this, faculty and student nurses need to acknowledge the fact that decisions must be made in spite of incomplete data collection. Seldom does real life allow one the luxury of collecting all of the relevant data before making any sort of decision; judgment based on knowledge and experience is relied upon. This is precisely the case in nursing:

informed judgment must be brought to bear in situations where a decision must be made before all the data is available. The skill to be taught then is the exercise of sound judgment (the educated guess) based on whatever facts are ready to hand. Student nurses need to learn this skill by seeing it in action, although equal care should be taken that a faculty member is not at their elbows continuously during this learning process; it then becomes the faculty member's judgment that is being used, and the student will be working to achieve approval from the teacher rather than working to solve the patient's presenting problem. In carefully controlled settings then, clinical decision making must be learned first by observing it and increasingly by practicing it.

Nurses who have been in practice for a few years have extraordinary skill in patient care decision making.

> I remember in my delivery room experience being awed by the old time delivery room nurses' knowledge of when to call a doctor. Not only could they predict the speed of an individual patient's dilation with unerring accuracy but they also knew how long it took each physician to travel from home to hospital or from office to hospital and manage to place the call at exactly the right time so that the doctor arrived precisely five minutes before delivery. Great skill went into making these judgments. In Primary Nursing, hopefully, that level of decision making sophistication can be directed at patient care decisions instead of physician care decisions.

Educational curriculum experts and students of learning theory can build opportunities for unsupervised clinical decision making experiences into the educational process, starting with basic and simple cases and gradually increasing the complexity to the greatest extent possible.

Clinical decision making in the hospital, whether by a student or experienced nurse, requires a knowledge of disease and a knowledge of human beings. Knowledge of the patient cannot be acquired in the classroom setting; it cannot even be acquired in short spurts of clinical exposure on a patient unit. Clinical decision making in nursing must be based on the nurse's firsthand knowledge of the sick person and this knowledge can best be acquired through the establishment and maintenance of a relationship over time. Thus, before students should be expected to make independent clinical decisions, the curriculum must be adjusted to permit them opportunities to establish therapeutic relationships with patients. This cannot be accomplished in a few hours a day, a few days a week; Primary Nursing requires that curricula be adjusted accordingly. Time must be allowed so that clinical decision making skills can be learned in a relatively independent fashion. Faculties have to learn to "let go" of their students just as head nurses have to learn to "let go" of their staff nurses when Primary Nursing is implemented. The art of "letting go" may actually help faculty members recognize the strength and weaknesses of the educational program better than any paper and pencil tests could.

Management of a number of cases simultaneously is another important skill needed in Primary Nursing. Setting priorities to get work done is a common enough concept in nursing service. Workload expansions and contractions inevitably occur without commensurate staffing adjustments, and since extra staff cannot be added to cover all such situations nurses need to learn how to decide which of their patients' needs will be met and which ones will not. Nurses may then feel less guilty about the fact that all patients do not receive all the care that they could simply because there are not adequate resources available. Nurses seem usually to be plagued with a tremendous sense of guilt about their inability to do everything for their patients. This is quickly transformed into anger and frustration, and enormous amounts of energy are wasted because of "short staffing." Nurses in hospitals today need to realize that there will never be as much help as they need or would like on their units and that the necessary priority decisions about how their time will be spent should only be made by them. Physician needs are often in competition with patient needs for nursing attention. Students should be taught that patient care needs come first and physician needs second. Once priorities have been set, nurses have to be realistic and stop feeling guilty about all the care they were unable to give, and learn instead to enjoy the accomplishments of delivering that care which is really essential.

The ability to establish, maintain and terminate the therapeutic relationship is another learning need made visible by Primary Nursing. Never a strong component of nursing education, this skill was ignored when this author was a student. We were taught not to get involved with our patients, to maintain a professional aloofness. Sister Madeline's work on commitment as an essential component of professional nursing helped pave the way for the kind of caring relationships that characterize the successful implementation of Primary Nursing [16]. The need for such relationship skills is more widely recognized now but the fact that many nurses are still very uncomfortable in this regard indicates that it should receive increased attention. No one is born with a complete and intact set of interpersonal skills; they must be learned and, until they are, it should be recognized that their lack is an educational lack, not an inadequacy in the nurse or in the system of Primary Nursing.

The Meaning of Clinical Specialization

For years the profession of nursing has been trying to identify logical parameters of clinical specialization around elements of nursing care rather than medical diagnoses. Nevertheless, clinical specialization in nursing still follows the medical model closely. Thus we have the cardiovascular nurse specialist, the diabetic nurse, the ostomy nurse, etc. On units where Primary Nursing is successfully implemented, a different delineation of nurse specialization often emerges spontaneously.

Before implementing the system on an oncology unit, I assumed the nurses' area of clinical expertise was a combination of knowledge about the care of patients with cancer who were undergoing chemotherapy and radiation therapy. After successful implementation I learned that the truly unique contribution that the nurses developed was in the area of caring for dying patients. Because of nursing's unique continuous presence, it was logical and sensible for nurses to become expert in helping patients and their families experience death in a supportive, therapeutic atmosphere.

On an OB unit, where I thought the nurses' area of expertise was postpartum care (breast feeding, bathing the baby and checking the episiotomy, etc.), I found that their real expertise lay in assisting patients to adjust to parenthood or enhancing their adjustment to the new family reality.

In other words, Primary Nursing, by focusing care on the person rather than on tasks, physicians, diseases or drugs, promotes a completely natural development of new definitions of clinical specialization. Careful analyses of these new roles need to be pursued by scholars and academicians in order to delineate, define and test the usefulness of new groupings of knowledge for nursing curricula.

The Power of Knowledge

The unique place of nursing in the health care delivery system is founded on the continuous knowledge that only the nurse can have of a patient, participating as she does in all of the events that affect him twenty-four hours a day, seven days a week. For example, a nurse is present when the patient is operated on, is present at 2:00 a.m. when he is consumed with apprehension about how his illness will affect his ability to provide for his family, is present at 7:00 a.m. when the dreaded diagnosis is delivered by the family physician and is present when the patient reacts to the pain of a spinal tap or the removal of dressings covering disfiguring surgery. The Primary Nurse is present and available to the patient during that time of particular closeness, the morning bath. She is present to listen, to hear, to interact with the person hospitalized for treatment. In some cases, nurses can know the hospitalized patient better than members of his own family, at least in terms of his hospitalization experience. The Primary Nursing system is designed to bring all of this knowledge together in one person who integrates and coordinates all aspects of the patient's care, making it possible to give care in a hospital that is as unified, personalized and humane as was the private duty nursing of years gone by.

None of the other health disciplines involved in the treatment of the hospitalized person has access to this broad spectrum of knowledge. They must all depend on the eyes and ears of the nursing staff for much of the information they require.

This kind of knowledge is powerful. It has heretofore received inadequate attention, but the slowly emerging realization of its value is helping to redefine the unique knowledge base upon which nursing as a profession can achieve a greater degree of autonomy. The Primary Nurse who appreciates and respects the importance of her knowledge will have a greater sense of self esteem and the true worth of her contribution to patient care. As this sense develops and is recognized both by herself and others, the Primary Nurse can claim her legitimate place beside other professionals and know the satisfaction of a dream finally achieved.

Addendum to Chapter Six

The concerns and issues discussed in Chapter Six remain today. The most fundamental challenge of Primary Nursing is autonomy. Without it, nursing remains a non-profession, regardless of the number of PhDs in the field. Nurse autonomy is the right and responsibility of the nurse to decide the amount, degree and kind of care the patient receives. The responsibility for this fundamental decision-making must lie with individuals willing and able to make competent decisions.

The challenge of preparing new nurses and developing nurses to make these decisions is as awesome today as it was twenty-five years ago. The main difference between then and now is that now both nurses and non-nurses recognize the importance of nurse autonomy.

However, many still find it convenient and reasonable to interpret this challenge in ways that obfuscate reality. Sometimes the challenge becomes an issue of basic educational levels rather than one of competence and empowerment. Sometimes obfuscation is related to workload and skill-mix issues. Sometimes it is based on organizational fears that nursing is getting too strong. Whatever the obfuscation, it has continued successfully to weaken the concept of nursing autonomy within and outside the profession.

Be all that as it is, the Primary Nurse is still the most logical person to teach clinical decision-making to students. This can best be done in short, on-the-unit sessions led by a skilled faculty member. A Socratic, or reflective questioning illuminates the complex clinical judgments Primary Nurses make in their daily practice.

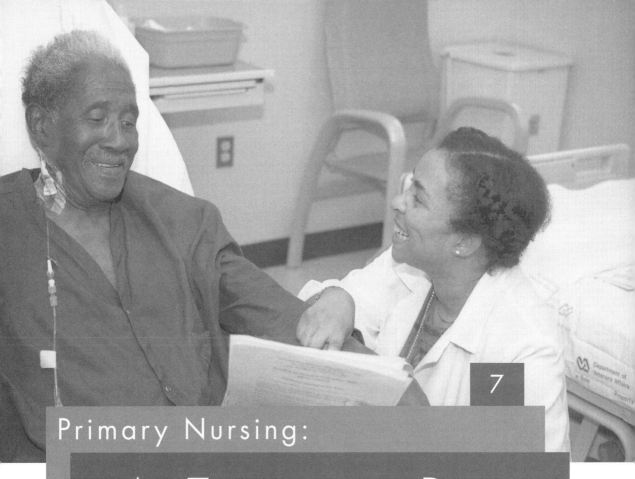

7

Primary Nursing:

A Turning Point

As I look back over the last thirty years, I see that the concept of Primary Nursing marked a cosmic shift in thinking about the delivery of professional nursing at the hospital bedside. Prior to its successful implementation on Station 32, the idea of nurses practicing professionally—with autonomy of decision-making about the degree, amount and kind of nursing care a patient would receive—was little more than a gleam in the eye of progressive thinkers, mostly academics who had little knowledge about how to make the necessary organization changes to create a realistic role for professional bedside nursing.

By the time we developed Primary Nursing, it was definitely an idea whose time had come. Others were also experimenting with changing the nursing care delivery system. Lydia Hall at Loeb Center created a whole new type of institution, a Nursing Center where total patient care was practiced with tremendous success. In many ways, I view our successful implementation as a matter of a correct convergence of important factors, rather than some uniquely creative venture, isolated from other efforts. Some of those important factors were an open-minded administration, deep frustration with the ways units were being managed and care being delivered, and the availability of experts in sociology, leadership, human dynamics and administration to advise and teach me the fundamentals of organizational dynamics.

In the beginning, several of us spent a great deal of time speaking about the work: The nurse manager, Diane Bartels; the CNS, Karen Ciske; the Hospital Administrator, Dave Preston; the Sociologist, Stan Williams; and several staff nurses, Colleen Person and Marjorie Page, to name a few. For most of them, time turned their attention away from this development and into other phases of their career. My career move was to a position as Director of Nursing at the Charles T. Miller hospital, where I followed an excellent long-tenured nurse leader, Thelma Dodds. She selected me as her successor partly because she saw the benefits of Primary Nursing and wanted that for the department she loved. Thus, I was able to learn about applying the decentralization within an administrative structure, as well how to structure a hospital-wide implementation from a leadership position. From an experience I had helping the Director of Nursing at St. Joseph's Hospital in St. Paul, I learned that I couldn't implement the system by management edict. Especially since the head nurses I inherited had twenty to thirty-five years experience running their floors from an authoritarian position. My career, therefore, kept me in the forefront of learning, thinking, speaking and writing about Primary Nursing from a variety of perspectives. Thus, I became the recognized expert regarding the implementation of Primary Nursing.

The successful implementation of decentralization principles within a hospital bureaucracy meant that forevermore the nursing profession knows it has a choice between task-based and relationship-based nursing care. We also know there are forces within the environment that impact the ease or difficulty in making that choice. The incredible pressure of using complex data in a highly technical activity often drives the caregiver's attention away from the human dimension of practice. The pendulum continues to swing: continuity of care becomes more challenging due to shortened lengths of stay coupled with 12-hour shift; with financial concerns dictating skill mix rather than patient acuity; and with CEOs, CNOs, and COOs philosophically uncomfortable giving bedside nurses authority over patient care. These factors and others mitigate sustained implementation. However, the pendulum swings. It is my opinion that the predominant factor in moving the pendulum from relationship-based practice is a change in administrative philosophy. New leadership seems to feel required to produce a shift in the fundamental orientation of the institution. When life was more static, conventional wisdom said a new administrator needed to paint the lobby to signal to employees that someone new was in the top office. Nowadays, the way that need is expressed is to change the administrative structure, move people around in the top positions, let a few people go and introduce budget cuts to improve the margins—the nonprofit term for profit. These changes often do more to reduce the commitment to relationship-based practice than anything else. It is just much safer to do the tasks—what can be measured and documented—and therefore rewarded and valued.

While Primary Nursing may conjure up unrealistic dreams, the principles of professional autonomous practice are continuously being reimplemented, sometimes under different names such as care coordinator and care manager. I believe it doesn't matter what the role is called. What matters is that the patients and their families know the name of the nurse who is responsible for managing their care over time. If that is known, then the system is in place, and the rest of the health care team, as well as the physician, will also know it. It is all about the nurse-patient relationship. The pendulum keeps swinging, and each time it returns to a relationship-based delivery system, patients receive the kind of coordinated and humane care they deserve.

Final Thoughts

Writing this in early October, 2001, the events of Sept 11, 2001 have changed the world in ways I can only imagine. One thing, however, seems certain. It seems that America will never again move unfettered into blind consumerism and commercial materialism. The terrorist attack on the World Trade Center and Washington, DC, brought our values of family, relationships and self-sacrifice to the forefront of our national consciousness. As never before since perhaps World War II, we see ourselves as a nation of basically good people who have enormous strength and capacity to do the right thing. When I think about how this change in national consciousness will affect hospitals and health care, I see more attention being paid to the fundamentals of nursing. I believe that if we can articulate the conceptual framework of our practice to the average person, as well as to the rest of the health care system, our profession will be accepted as it never was before Sept. 11. We will never again have to defend the value of an unregulated, undocumented interpersonal interaction of caring. However, as a profession, we still must find our voice to speak the truth about nursing care.

Commonly Asked Questions about Primary Nursing Answered with Common Sense

Does the Primary Nurse Always Work the Day Shift?

No, not necessarily. Since the day shift is usually more heavily staffed than either evenings or nights, it stands to reason that the majority of Primary Nurses will be assigned to work days. Also, the day nurse has the greatest opportunity to maintain good communication links with the other members of the health team (most of whom, for some reason, also work only the day shift).

In hospitals where there is shift rotation, Primary Nurse/patient assignments will usually remain intact when a nurse rotates from days to evenings. The logic is that the nurse can continue to maintain a therapeutic relationship with the patient even though she is working evenings (the patient is awake and can communicate) and that the integrity of the relationship is very important. Admittedly, the Primary Nurse may have to compromise the direct communication element of the system, but that compromise is of secondary importance to the maintenance of the relationship. When a Primary Nurse rotates to nights, however, if she still has primary patients (she would usually not be assigned new patients prior to night rotation) they might well be reassigned to one of the day or evening nurses.

In hospitals which have permanent shift assignments, evening and night nurses can have Primary Nurse assignments, but their caseload is usually smaller than that of day nurses. The decision about which patients to assign to permanent evening and night nurses ought to focus on patient needs. Some patients seem to require the most sophisticated level of nursing on the 3 to 11 shift after family members go home. Other patients have trouble sleeping nights and require the most thoughtful attention on that tour of duty. These and other such considerations should be taken into account in making evening and night assignments. From a staffing standpoint it is seldom, if ever, necessary to assign the night nurse a Primary Nurse caseload; this type of assignment should be made when it makes sense for a particular patient, rather than as a routine.

A word about nurses who are not Primary Nurses. Special care must be taken to avoid the development of yet another second-class citizenship issue in nursing, this one between Primary Nurses and all other staff members. Those who are not Primary Nurses ought not be made to feel that they are less worthy in any sense. The worth of a contribution must not be based on titles. A smoothly operating floor works only because of the contributions of all the staff working together from new graduate to ward clerk, from Nurses' Aide to Primary Nurse. Individuals must be valued because of their contributions to the over-all system; no one should feel diminished in stature because of Primary Nursing.

Who Should Assign the Patient?
What About the Idea of Nurses Selecting Their Own Patients?

The assignment of a Primary Nurse to a patient is usually made within 24 hours after admission. While the assignment decision is not usually difficult or time-consuming to make, it is complex, involving consideration of many factors. The head nurse as manager has ultimate responsibility for this function as a part of her overall duties of resource allocation. In many instances the Primary Nurse assignment decision becomes a matter of staff nurse decision making, which is based on clinical interests, workload, ability, needs of the patients, etc. *It doesn't matter* if the Primary Nurse assignment is made by the head nurse, a charge nurse, a specially designated staff nurse, or each Primary Nurse. The head nurse can choose to delegate this responsibility as long as the staff member designated uses good judgment. If problems of poor judgment arise, though, the head nurse has the ultimate responsibility for resolving them.

Does the Patient Have Anything to Say About Who His/her Primary Nurse Is?

Yes, an important factor in the Primary Nurse assignment is the patient's right to participate in the decision making process. Since most nurses are not initially known by the newly admitted patients, participation at the point of admission is usually limited to patients who have been previously hospitalized on the unit. If at any time during a patient's hospitalization he or she expresses the desire to change Primary Nurses, or expresses an inability to relate well with his Primary Nurse, reassignment should be made quickly and with impunity. Nurses frequently ask me how to handle the situation in which they do not get along with the patient they have been assigned. My answer is always that you should be able to request reassignment without its becoming an issue and the same is true when a patient does not get along with the nurse. Extreme care must be taken to ensure that a patient requesting reassignment to a different Primary Nurse is in no way punished or negatively treated by any of the staff. In any situation where the patient has an opportunity to know the staff members, such as small community hospitals or in cases where the patient is being re-hospitalized, every effort should be made to permit the patient to choose his own Primary Nurse as long as his selection is therapeutically effective.

How Does Primary Nursing Work for the Chronically Ill
Patient Who Is Hospitalized for an Extended Period of Time?

This question usually leads to a more widespread issue regarding nurse/patient assignments: What do you do if a nurse gets tired of a patient or is not, for any reason, getting along with him? Since the essence of Primary Nursing is the establishment of a therapeutic relationship, failure to achieve or maintain such a relationship is adequate justification for reassignment. This is a completely normal situation which should be handled without chastising either the patient or the nurse.

Chronically ill patients are not necessarily "problem patients." Many nurses find they offer an especially rewarding type of challenge. However, during long term hospitalization, two types of reassignment situations may occur. First, a Primary Nurse may need to be relieved of daily care activities once in a while. This should be done in a matter of fact manner. Second, a nurse may need to be relieved temporarily or permanently on her Primary Nurse responsibilities. This too should be accomplished in a matter of fact manner, making sure the patient understands the change without being made to feel rejected by the Primary Nurse.

Do All Patients Need a Primary Nurse?

Yes. Rather than considering the question on a need basis, I prefer to answer on a "right" basis. I believe all patients have a right to know who is making decisions regarding their nursing care and who is "in charge" of it. When patients have the names of the responsible physician and the responsible nurse managing their cases, true accountability for hospital care can be established.

Because Primary Nursing is incredibly difficult to implement in settings where immature attitudes prevail, I do not feel it will be available to all patients in the foreseeable future. However, wherever the system is implemented, I believe all patients in that setting (hospital, or floor, or patient care division) have an equal right to know the names of the nurses responsible for their care. Thus, *I feel it is unfair and unwise to have some patients with a Primary Nurse and others without one in a single unit*.

How About a Very Short Term Patient—One Who Is Hospitalized Just Overnight?

Since that patient will be receiving some nursing care during his short stay, I see no reason why he should not know the name of the nurse responsible for that care. Someone will be making some kind of decisions. The question is whether or not the patient need know who that person is when he is in so briefly, and the answer is still "yes." It may not be necessary to have a nursing care plan or discharge plan for the short term patient, but Primary Nursing is visible responsibility for decision making, not the existence of elaborate care plans.

What Is an Associate Primary Nurse?
Should an Associate Nurse Always Take Care of the Same Primary Nurse's Patients Each Day?

The words "associate nurse" were originally used to describe the role of the staff member who took care of the patient when the Primary Nurse was off duty, and it is in this sense that I have used them. In some hospitals, however, the words have been used as a job description rather than a shift role assignment. I do not agree with the use of "Associate Primary Nurse" as a job title for many reasons, not the least of which is that it creates another level in an already too-many-layered hierarchy.

The system of Primary Nursing builds in continuity of care through the Primary Nurse who takes care of her own patient each shift she works and who leaves instructions for others to follow. Some hospitals have tried to enhance that continuity by maintaining continuity of the associate nurse/patient assignment. The logistics of accomplishing this are awkward but if it can be managed without inordinately complex planning then care must be taken to prevent excessive isolation among station personnel. In Primary Nursing staff members develop a much more profound knowledge of fewer patients, but it is still

83

important that all staff members have at least a general idea of what is going on with all the patients. I find it is helpful to think of Primary Nurse, Associate Primary Nurse, or charge nurse as ad hoc role assignments any experienced registered nurse should be expected to be able to perform, rather than thinking of them as position titles. This increases the flexibility of utilization of the staff. Then Associate Primary Nurse assignments can be handled by different individuals depending on the circumstances on a shift. Continuity is maintained through the Primary Nurse's instructions.

What Is the Role of the Clinical Specialist?

Without getting into the controversy about educational preparation, I will define clinical specialist as one who has a greater scope and breadth of clinical knowledge in a particular field than that of the average staff nurse. Using this definition, the contribution of the clinical specialist is made whenever a staff nurse is caring for a patient whose care needs require clinical knowledge at the specialist level. The Primary Nurse requests a consult from the specialist who makes an assessment and leaves recommendations. The Primary Nurse must be free to accept or reject these recommendations since she has superior knowledge of the total patient. If she decides to reject the specialist's recommendations she should be expected to be able to explain her rationale for doing so to the head nurse who is ultimately responsible for the quality of care administered to all the patients on the unit. The logical role then for clinical specialists in Primary Nursing is that of expert consultant. They can also make a significant contribution as Primary Nurses themselves for patients with extremely complex care requirements, or as co-Primary Nurses to back up a staff nurse in a complicated clinical situation. In addition, the clinical specialist ought to be available to teach nurses whatever they need to know in order to continue improving patient care.

Should the Head Nurse Take a Primary Nurse Assignment?

It doesn't matter. Many head nurses have found after implementing this system that they have time to manage a small caseload, usually one or two patients. By doing so, they can share in the dynamic rewards of being a nurse for a sick person and can also provide a powerful role model. Sometimes head nurses prefer to be Associate Primary Nurses and use this opportunity to strengthen a new nurse's knowledge base, assess her learning, and so on. Some head nurses function as a Primary Nurse at times, as an Associate at others and as neither when their head nurse responsibilities require their full attention. However, some head nurses decide never to take a patient assignment, either as Associate or as Primary Nurse. If they are able to establish an effective teacher/clinician/leader role using other techniques, having caseloads of their own is not vitally important.

Appendix B
Notes on Developing a Professional Practice Model

Excerpt from *The Professional Practice Model: A Guide for Implementation*, edited by Mary Koloroutis

The nurse-patient relationship is the cornerstone of professional nursing practice and fundamental to a care delivery model known for excellence. There is universal agreement among nurses that inherent in their relationships with patients and families is a privileged trust which they must hold sacred. Nurses voice a fierce commitment to the values of caring, advocacy, collaboration, safety, and seeking what is in the best interest of the patients and families they serve. Nurses are also expressing frustration in trying to live these values in daily practice within the context of existing care delivery models and the challenges of the health care system. You have decided to move into action and to transform your current care delivery system into a professional practice model that supports your ability to live what matters most to you, your colleagues, and the patients and families you serve.

To "*transform*" means "*to change the condition*" of what currently exists. Such transformation, unfortunately, doesn't just happen. Transforming nursing practice through the design and implementation of a professional practice model has three requirements:

1. It takes leaders and staff at all levels of the organization with a shared vision and commitment to caring for patients;
2. It requires a methodology to guide the way;
3. It takes impeccable communication, collaboration, and follow through.

The creative plans that evolve through this work can result in new efficient and effective ways of providing nursing care that enhances satisfaction for nurses and patients and their families. This implementation guide provides background information regarding professional practice and care delivery models and guidance for each of the six phases of the transformation process: preparation, structure, planning, review and support, implementation, and continuous improvement.

Any group implementing a new model needs information, support, and guidance. Meet with your nursing leaders and colleagues to develop a shared vision of what you would like Professional Nursing Practice to be on your unit. Review your current care delivery system to identify opportunities for change. Refresh and renew your understanding of professional practice through individual reading and group discussion.

(Bibliographies, books and videotapes are available through Creative HealthCare Resources to support the work of the committee.)

Definitions of the Nature & Scope of Professional Nursing Practice

"…nursing is to have charge of the personal health of somebody and what nursing has to do is to put the patient in the best condition for nature to act upon him…"
Notes on Nursing: What It Is and What It Is Not
Florence Nightingale, 1859

Professional nursing exists to provide compassionate care to individuals and their loved ones. Nursing is one segment of a complex, interdependent health care delivery system. The focus of nursing practice is to help people maintain health, effect healing, cope during times of stress and suffering, and to experience a dignified and peaceful death. This is achieved through clinical knowledge and proficiency and a profound understanding of the human condition.

The American Nurses' Association (ANA) defines nursing as *"the diagnosis and treatment of human responses to actual or potential health problems"* and clarifies the scope of nursing practice through four defining characteristics: 1) Boundary, 2) Intersections, 3) Core, and 4) Dimensions. The source of the definitions of these characteristics presented below is *A Social Policy Statement, ANA, 1980.* The implications are from the work of Creative HealthCare Management.

Boundary

Definition: Webster's defines boundary as *"something that indicates or fixes a limit or extent."* According to ANA, the boundary for nursing, as is true for all professions, is dynamic rather than static. It expands outward in response to changing needs, demands and capacities of society. As the boundary changes, the other three characteristics, intersections, core, and dimensions, begin to change.

Implications: It is essential that professional boundaries be clearly articulated for successful role implementation. It is the responsibility of each individual within their professional role to understand the nature and extent of their responsibility, authority, and accountability (RAA.) Within an organization RAA must be articulated and negotiated with the professional nursing staff. RAA for professional nurses are defined through licensure, professional standards, and position descriptions. Responsibility, authority and accountability are defined on the next page:

> **Responsibility**—The clear and specific allocation of work duties. It is a two-way process. Responsibility is achieved when there is allocation and acceptance in conjunction with ownership and action. Responsibility is visibly given. Acceptance of responsibility answers the question: "Am I doing what I agreed to do?"

Authority—The right/freedom to act in the areas where one is given and accepts responsibility. Levels of authority need to be clear and are based on the scope of the situation (problem to be resolved) and competency of the individual or group. Authority answers the question: "Do I have the knowledge and ability to make this decision or take this action for which I have accepted responsibility?"

Accountability—The obligation to account for one's responsibilities through evaluating the outcomes of one's decisions and actions in order to direct future efforts. Accountability answers the questions: "Have I done what I said I would do? What was the result? What have I learned? What follow-up is needed?" All nurses are ethically and legally accountable for actions taken in the course of their practice.

Intersection

Definition: Intersection means to *"meet or cross at a point."* Nurses intersect with other health professionals in the care of patients. These relationships, when effective and healthy, are driven by a mutual focus and desire to serve the best interests of patients and families. All of the health care professions share the same overall mission and purpose, have access to the same published research and health care literature, and acknowledge the need to work cooperatively and interdependently for quality results.

Implications: It is well-known that the number one indicator for safe, quality care delivery is effective and respectful teamwork. Teams that have clearly defined responsibility, authority, and accountability have the functional foundation for healthy working relationships. The nurse must balance multiple relationships to effectively coordinate care. First, there is the primary relationship with the patient and family. This relationship drives care delivery through developing a mutually determined and well-communicated plan of care. Second, the nurse-physician relationship is fundamental. Patients and families are safely cared for when there is ongoing communication and collaboration between the nurse and physician. When this relationship is not clear, respectful, and proactive, patient safety is compromised. Third, the nurse relates to all members of the health care team to assure the patient and family receive coordinated and essential services. These members include anyone within the organization that supports and or delivers care to patients and families. Effective, quality care delivery is contingent upon healthy, interdependent relationships between all members of the health care team.

Characteristics of healthy interdependent relationships are:

Trust—this ranges from the expectation that a team member will demonstrate *"trustworthiness"* to the belief that a team member can do the work they are there to do (*"functional trust."*) Trustworthy people are able to develop a trust relationship which comes from having a balance in character (integrity and maturity) and competence (technical, critical thinking, interpersonal).

Mutual Respect—this signifies that the relationships have moved beyond titles, positions, educational level to an appreciation for one another, for who they are and for their contribution. Respect is given, regardless of external criteria.

Consistent, Visible Support—this is built on a foundation of trust and mutual respect and means that individuals and groups continually strive to achieve win-win relationships. It does not mean having the same opinion; it does mean achieving results through active and respectful communication, problem-solving, and learning.

Open and Honest Communication—good and clear communication starts with each individual owning their part or responsibility. The primary goal is to listen and increase understanding. A key factor is to listen and speak directly and truthfully with the person or people effected.

Core

Definition: Core means central or foundational part. The core of nursing includes those essential characteristics that represent the foundation or art and science of nursing care.

The core characteristics of professional nursing practice are provided through relationships and grounded in privileged intimacy—a "laying-on-of hands" practice in which nurses have access to the body of another person in carrying out assessments, comfort care, and treatments. There is a basic commitment to respecting the worth and dignity of people with a profound regard for humanity.

Caring is a primary and ethical obligation. It includes independent nursing acts, delegated actions based on the medical plan of care and interdependent actions based on the interdisciplinary treatment plan.

Implications: A successful professional practice model is one in which these core characteristics of nursing practice are the foundation and are achieved through the design of the nursing care delivery system. Nurses understand and value the nursing activities of professional practice and the system is designed to support these activities. There needs to be careful consideration regarding the scope of responsibility, authority, and accountability for all members of the health care team. Work assignments need to be consistent with the appropriate scope of practice and the level of competency for each team member. Patient assignments are made with the commitment to safeguarding the professional nurse-patient relationship.

Dimensions

Definition: A definition of dimensions in Webster's is, *"one of the elements or factors making up a complete entity."* Dimensions for professional nursing practice are those elements that further describe, enhance, and/or deepen the meaning, purpose and scope of nursing care delivery. These would include, but not be limited to: descriptions of core values and beliefs (philosophy); ethical principles or statements; scientific theories, nursing theories, research findings, professional standards; organization-specific documents i.e. mission/values statements and job descriptions; and regulatory agency standards/ requirements (i.e. JCAHO, HCFA).

Implications: Dimensions connect a professional practice model and the nursing care delivery system with the broader aspects of health care delivery. There are many dimensions that are universal, i.e. ANA standards, codes of ethics, scientific theories. Also, realistically, the JCAHO and HCFA standards are universal dimensions for care delivery within hospitals in the United States. By specifying dimensions that inform your practice and by designing your care delivery model to meet standards within these dimensions, you achieve a knowledge-based and proactive system of care.

Review of Basic Nursing Practice

The first step in understanding and evaluating the changes that will occur in the implementation of the professional practice model is to review the basics of nursing practice. The steering committee and the unit practice committee may add to these basics in ways that are compatible with the principles of the organization-specific model. The following chart summarizes the basics of nursing and the activities carried out in support of those elements. (Adapted from the work of Marie Manthey)

Basics of Practice: Specific Nursing Activities

1. Assess the patient and family needs
   a. Conduct a nursing assessment and determine nursing needs/diagnoses through listening to the person's story, interviews and review of records
   b. Develop an individualized plan of nursing care with the patient/family
2. Implement the medical orders:
   a. assess orders to assure these match the needs and desires of the patient
   b. evaluate the effect of the medical orders
3. Continuously assess, taking action as needed
4. Communicate the medical and nursing plan to others (assistive staff and multidisciplinary colleagues)
5. Manage and deliver the nursing care associated with the patient's medical and nursing diagnosis
   a. Establish a therapeutic relationship with the patient
   b. Continuously assess, monitor and prevent complications
   c. Administer and evaluate medical and nursing treatments
   d. Delegate activities of nursing care appropriately
   e. Revise the nursing diagnoses and plans as the patients status changes
6. Communicate and coordinate care during the patients length of stay with others who are interacting with the patient
   a. Provide information about the patient in report and care conferences
   b. Conduct problem solving to resolve issues identified
   c. Coordinate with multidisciplinary colleagues.
7. Coordinate the patient transfer or discharge
   a. Teach aspects of care that will need to be carried out upon discharge to patient and/or family members
   b. Communicate care needs and approaches to others who will care for the patient after discharge
   c. Communicate with case manager or discharge planner

In functional, total patient care or team nursing models, many of the basic elements are attended to by the nurse manager, charge nurse or team leader. In a professional practice model, these responsibilities are assumed by the nurse at the bedside in relationship with the patient over time.

References

1. This and other quotations in this chapter are taken from the student records on the Connecticut Training School, New Haven, for the years 1890 to 1910.
2. Kramer, M. *Reality Shock*. St. Louis: Mosby, 1974.
3. Gelinas, A. *Nursing and Nursing Education*. New York: The Commonwealth Fund, 1946. p. 9.
4. Brown, E.L. *Nursing for the Future*. New York: Russell Sage Foundation, 1944.
5. *Towards Quality in Nursing Report of the Surgeon General's Consultant Group in Nursing*. Washington, DC: United States Public Health Service, 1963. p. 15.
6. Ibid.
7. Kramer, ibid.
8. American Nursing Association, Committee on Education. ANA's first position paper on education for nursing, *Am. J. Nurs.* 65:106, 1965.
9. Aydelotte, M.K. and Tever, M.E. *An Investigation of the Relation Between Nursing Activity and Patient Welfare*. Iowa City: State University of Iowa, 1960.
10. United States Public Health Service, Division of Nursing. *How to Study Activities on a Patient Unit* (rev. ed.). Washington, DC: US Government Printing Office (PHS Publication No. 570), 1964.
11. Ibid.
12. Personal communication by group of nurses doing Primary Nursing at Yale-New Haven Hospital interviewed by author during 1979.
13. Ibid.
14. Barrett, J. *Word Management and Teaching*. London: Appleton-Century-Crofts, 1949.
15. Goodman, P. *People or Personnel: Decentralizing and the Mixed System*. Toronto: Random House, 1965.
16. Vaillot, Sister Madeline Clemence. *Existentialism; A Philosophy of Commitment, Am. J. Nurs.* 66:38, 1966

Index

Components of a
Relationship-Based Care Delivery System

Leaders know the vision, act with purpose, remove barriers, and consistently hold patients, families and staff as their highest priority.

Teamwork requires a group of diverse members from all disciplines and departments to define and embrace a shared purpose and to work together to fulfill that purpose.

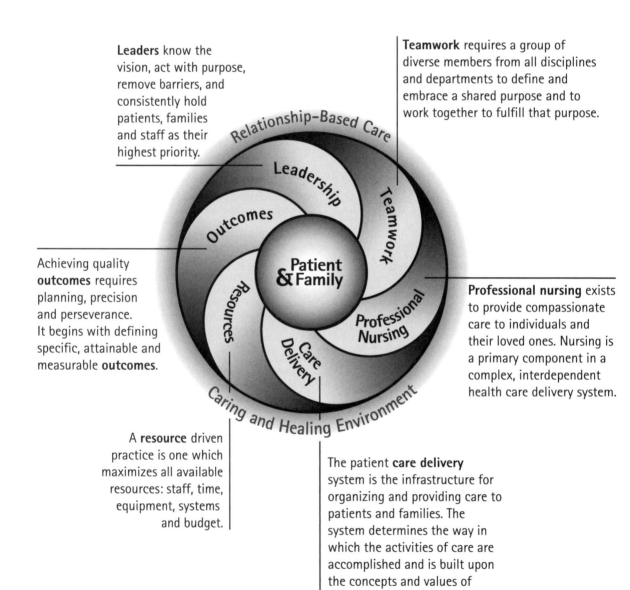

Achieving quality **outcomes** requires planning, precision and perseverance. It begins with defining specific, attainable and measurable **outcomes**.

Professional nursing exists to provide compassionate care to individuals and their loved ones. Nursing is a primary component in a complex, interdependent health care delivery system.

A **resource** driven practice is one which maximizes all available resources: staff, time, equipment, systems and budget.

The patient **care delivery** system is the infrastructure for organizing and providing care to patients and families. The system determines the way in which the activities of care are accomplished and is built upon the concepts and values of professional nursing practice.

Consulting Services from Creative Health Care Management:
A Critical Step in a Successful Relationship-Based Care Implementation.

Relationship-Based Care (RBC)

is an adaptation of Primary Nursing for the current state of health care with short-term patients, part-time nurses, and 12-hour shifts. RBC provides the map and highlights the most direct routes to achieve world-class care and service to patients and families in your organization. Organizations who have implemented this model report an increase in patient satisfaction and loyalty, an increase in staff and physician satisfaction and a more resource conscious and efficient work environment.

Here are some of the ways we can help you implement Relationship-Based Care:

- **Education Session**. How does RBC work on individual units and system wide? What outcomes can be expected? (Half day or one day)

- **Design Day**. A customized design for your organization and the infrastructure needed to support the implementation of the RBC model. (One day)

- **Appreciative Inquiry Organizational Assessment**. Identifies organizational strengths and desired outcomes. (One to two days)

- **Reigniting the Spirit of Caring**. An inspirational/educational experience to enhance awareness about the different dimensions of caring: caring for self, colleagues, patients and their families. (Three days)

- **Relationships at the Point of Care.** Designed for employees working directly with the patient, this program teaches effective leadership qualities, human dynamics concepts, and effective communication skills. (One day)

- **Leadership at the Point of Care**. Provides clinical leaders the knowledge and skills to create a healing environment for participants and colleagues. (Three days)

- **Inspirational Caring.** Helps create an appreciative and supportive environment to reflect and dialogue about the meaning and purpose of caring for people within our health care organizations. (One day)

- **Relationship-Based Care Practicum**. A practical five day intensive to provide RBC Project Leaders with the clarity and competence essential for assembling a collaborative team of change leaders. Also a chance to share strategies, ideas and challenges with others implementing Relationship-Based Care. (Five days)

The Relationship-Based Care Practicum
Training for Leaders and Team Members

Leading the Change to Relationship-Based Care

Sharing the RBC concept with peers and employees, helping managers understand its benefits, and making it a success in your organization is a true challenge. Implementing what matters most in a complex environment requires persistence and strategic knowledge and skills. We know these skills and knowledge can be taught, learned, and applied to any organizational environment. Whether you're a new or experienced RBC Leader, this program will help give you the direction you need to make RBC succeed at your organization. Join us in taking RBC to another level. Enjoy learning and sharing ideas and strategies with other RBC participant teams throughout the country.

The Relationship-Based Care Practicum has been developed specifically to help with the challenges you face in implementing Relationship-Based Care. This practical five day course will provide RBC Leaders with the clarity and competence essential for assembling a collaborative team of change leaders. The program blends a variety of experiential methodologies to develop competencies, integrate learning relative to RBC, and design customized strategies and outcomes in your individual organizations. The experiential methodologies such as dialogue, circle and reflection, appreciative inquiry, and action learning will ensure that participants are actively involved in the experience and apply their learning through presentations and group discussions.

For more information visit:
www.relationshipbasedcare.com

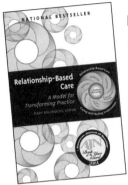

Relationship-Based Care:
A Model for Transforming Practice

Mary Koloroutis, Editor

The result of Creative Health Care Management's 25 years experience in transforming patient care, this book provides health care leaders with practical approaches for transforming their care delivery system into one that is patient and family centered and built on the power of relationships. *Relationship-Based Care* provides a practical framework for addressing current challenges and is intended to benefit health care organizations in which commitment to care and service to patients is strong and focused. It will also prove useful in organizations searching for solutions to complex struggles with patient, staff and physician dissatisfaction; difficulty recruiting and retaining and developing talented staff members; conflicted work relationships and related quality issues. Now a national bestseller with over 30,000 copies sold and a winner of the *American Journal of Nursing* Book of the Year Award.

Softcover, 288 pages. (2004) $34.95
ISBN 13: 978-1-886624-19-1

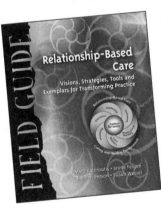

Relationship-Based Care Field Guide:
Visions, Strategies, Tools and Exemplars
for Transforming Practice

Mary Koloroutis, Jayne Felgen, Colleen Person, Susan Wessel

This follow-up title to the award winning, national bestseller *Relationship-Based Care: A Model for Transforming Practice*, shows readers how Relationship-Based Care transforms the culture of care delivery – organization wide and at the bedside. Written as a field guide, this book will inspire those who are working on the critical relationships that deliver superior patient care.

Using a unique framework centered around inspiration, infrastructure, education and evidence (I_2E_2), the editors compile stories and experiences of real executives, managers, and front-line care givers implementing Relationship-Based Care nation wide and around the world. *Relationship-Based Care Field Guide: Visions, Strategies, Tools and Exemplars for Transforming Practice* is an essential resource for anyone wanting to implement Relationship-Based Care.

Softcover, 736 pages. (2007) $99.00
ISBN 13: 978-1-886624-23-8

107

For more information visit:
www.relationshipbasedcare.com

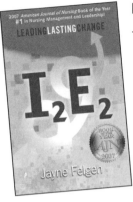

I₂E₂: Leading Lasting Change
Jayne Felgen

In *I₂E₂: Leading Lasting Change*, Jayne Felgen shares her in-depth, practical and elegantly simple formula for inspiring and leading real change at all levels of any organization. *I₂E₂* is not a step-by-step guide to re-creating the new west business model; rather, it is a new way of embracing change. Leaders learn to organize the whole process, from shared vision to detailed changes in infrastructure. *I₂E₂* is a simple and elegant formula for initiating and sustaining lasting change over time.

Softcover, 181 pages. (2007) $24.95
ISBN 13: 978-1-886624-12-2

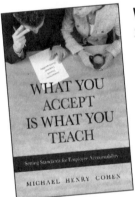

What You Accept is What You Teach:
Setting Standards for Employee Accountability
Michael H. Cohen

What You Accept is What You Teach offers practical advice for managers on how to hold employees accountable for a strong work ethic, intrinsic motivation, a positive attitude and constructive conduct toward customers and co-workers. It describes a leader's rights and responsibilities relative to maintaining standards for teamwork, customer service and technical competence. This book includes tools to effectively confront and set limits with employees who demonstrate counter-productive and passive-aggressive behaviors that raise havoc with group morale. This is the perfect "how to" guide for navigating the maze of challenging employee communication and performance.

Softcover, 191 pages. (2007) $16.00
ISBN 13: 978-1-886624-76-4

ORDER FORM

1. Call toll-free 800.264.3246 and use your Visa, Mastercard or American Express or a company purchase order

2. Fax your order to: 952.854.1866

3. Mail your order with pre-payment or company purchase order to:

   Creative Health Care Management
   1701 American Blvd East, Suite 1
   Minneapolis, MN 55425
   Attn: Resources Department

CREATIVE

HEALTH CARE

MANAGEMENT

4. Order Online at: www.chcm.com

Product	Price	Quantity	Subtotal	TOTAL
B240 *The Practice of Primary Nursing, 2nd Edition*	$19.95			
B510 *Relationship-Based Care: A Model for Transforming Practice*	$34.95			
B600 *Relationship-Based Care Field Guide*	$99.00			
B560 *I_2E_2: Leading Lasting Change*	$24.95			
B558 *What You Accept is What You Teach*	$16.00			
Shipping Costs: 1 book - $6.50, 2-9 - $7.50, 10 or more - $10.00 *Call for express rates*				
Order TOTAL				

Need more than one copy? We have quantity discounts available.

Quantity Discounts (Books Only)		
10–24 = *10% off*	25–99 = *25% off*	100 or more = *35% off*

Payment Methods: ☐ Credit Card   ☐ Check   ☐ Purchase Order PO# _____

Credit Card	Number			Expiration	AVS (3 digits)
Visa / Mastercard / American Express	–	–	–	/	
Cardholder address (if different from below):		Signature:			

Customer Information	
Name:	
Title:	
Company:	
Address:	
City, State, Zip:	
Daytime Phone:	
Email:	

Satisfaction guarantee: If you are not satisfied with your purchase, simply return the products within 30 days for a full refund. For a free catalog of all our products, visit www.chcm.com or call 800.264.3246.